RENAL DIET

Guide To Manage Phosphorus Intake in Order to Manage and Avoid Kidney Disease

(Easy Recipes for Healthy Kidneys)

Nigel Lozano

Published by Alex Howard

© **Nigel Lozano**

All Rights Reserved

Renal Diet: Guide To Manage Phosphorus Intake in Order to Manage and Avoid Kidney Disease (Easy Recipes for Healthy Kidneys)

ISBN 978-1-989891-88-9

Legal & Disclaimer

The information contained in this book is not designed to replace or take the place of any form of medicine or professional medical advice. The information in this book has been provided for educational and entertainment purposes only.

TABLE OF CONTENTS

PART 1.. 1

INTRODUCTION 2

CHAPTER 1: THE 21 DAYS MEAL PLAN 18

DAY 1 18

BREAKFAST RECIPE.. 18

QUESADILLAS WITH PEARS 18

LUNCH RECIPE... 19

CHICKEN AND SWEET POTATO STIR FRY 19

DINNER 20

SEA BASS WITH BASIL-TOMATO TOPPING 20

SNACKS 21

CHOCOLATE BEET CAKE... 21

DAY 2... 21

BREAKFAST.. 22

OPEN-FACED BAGEL BREAKFAST SANDWICH 22

LUNCH... 23

SWORDFISH AND CITRUS SALSA DELIGHT............................ 23

DINNER 24

AROMATIC CHICKEN AND CABBAGE STIR-FRY 24

SNACKS 25

VEGETABLE LENTIL SOUP 25

DAY 3... 26

BREAKFAST.. 26

PEACH BERRY PARFAIT... 26

LUNCH **27**

RED COLESLAW WITH APPLE 27

DINNER **27**

CHICKEN SOUP WITH KALE AND SWEET POTATOES 27

SNACKS **29**

HERBED CABBAGE STEW 29
DAY 4 30

BREAKFAST **30**

EGG IN THE HOLE 30

LUNCH **31**

LEMON-HERB CHICKEN 31

DINNER **32**

CHICKEN CHOW MEIN 32

SNACKS **33**

CHICKEN PHO 33
DAY 5 34

BREAKFAST **34**

BROCCOLI BASIL QUICHE 34

LUNCH **35**

HERB-GARLIC SAUCE OVER PAN FRIED FISH 35

DINNER **36**

PARSNIP AND PEAR SOUP 37

SNACKS **37**

ROASTED ROOT VEGETABLES 37
DAY 6 38
BREAKFAST 38

LUNCH **41**

Roasted Cauliflower with Mixed Greens Salad..41

DINNER **42**

Persian Chicken 42

SNACKS **43**

Scrumptious Apple Bars 43
Day 7...44

BREAKFAST..**44**

Breakfast Banana Delight 44

LUNCH..**45**

Creole Jambalaya 45

DINNER **46**

Garlic Cauliflower Rice...46

SNACKS **47**

Thai-Style Eggplant Dip 47
Day 8...48

BREAKFAST..**48**

Pear, Chicken and Almond Garden Salad 48

LUNCH..**49**

Celery and Arugula Salad..49

DINNER **50**

Chicken Breast and Bok Choy in Parchment 50

SNACKS **51**

Pineapple Raspberry Parfaits 51
Day 9...51

BREAKFAST..**51**

Egg And Veggie Muffins 51

LUNCH... **52**

ROASTED BEET SALAD 52

DINNER **53**

INDIAN CHICKEN CURRY 53

SNACKS **54**

SIMPLE ROASTED BROCCOLI 54

DAY 10... 55

BREAKFAST... **55**

POPPY SEED-LEMON DRESSING ON WINTER FRUIT SALAD 55

LUNCH... **56**

SUMMER PASTA SALAD WITH WHITE WINE VINAIGRETTE........................... 56

DINNER **57**

THAI-STYLE CHICKEN CURRY 57

SNACKS **58**

ROASTED RED PEPPER HUMMUS... 58

DAY 11... 59

BREAKFAST... **59**

BAKED OATMEAL WITH APPLE SPICE FLAVOR.............................. 59

LUNCH... **60**

EASY BAKED SHEPHERD'S PIE 60

DINNER **61**

CHICKPEAS SOUP MOROCCAN STYLE 61

SNACKS **62**

ALMOND WALNUT GRANOLA 62

DAY 12... 63

BREAKFAST... **63**

Sandwich with Spinach and Tuna Salad 63

LUNCH.. **64**

Quick Thai Chicken and Vegetable Curry 64

DINNER **65**

Chicken Satay with Peanut Sauce... 66

SNACKS **67**

Vegetable Couscous 67
Day 13... 68

BREAKFAST... **68**

Quinoa, Cilantro and Cranberry Salad 68

LUNCH.. **69**

Mexican Baked Beans and Rice 69

DINNER **70**

Turkey Meatballs and Spaghetti in Garlic Sauce 70

SNACKS **71**

Pumpkin Walnut Cookie 71
Day 14... 72

BREAKFAST... **72**

Pasta with Parmesan Broccoli Sauce 72

LUNCH.. **73**

Pear and Watercress Salad... 73

DINNER **74**

Chicken Stir-Fry 74

SNACKS **75**

Collard Salad Rolls with Peanut Dipping Sauce... 75
Day 15... 77

BREAKFAST.. 77

SLOW COOKED BREAKFAST OATMEAL... 77

LUNCH.. 78

CHICKEN, CHARRED TOMATO AND BROCCOLI SALAD 78

DINNER 79

BAKED HERBED CHICKEN.. 79

SNACKS 80

DELICIOUSLY GOOD TUNA DIP 80

DAY 16.. 81

BREAKFAST.. 81

BUCKWHEAT PANCAKES 81

LUNCH.. 82

BULGUR AND BROCCOLI SALAD 82

DINNER 83

SWISS CHARD, WHITE BEAN & PASTA SOUP 83

SNACKS 85

CHOCO-CHIP COOKIES WITH WALNUTS AND OATMEAL............................. 85

DAY 17.. 86

BREAKFAST.. 86

CEREAL WITH CRANBERRY-ORANGE TWIST 86

LUNCH.. 87

LASAGNA ROLLS IN MARINARA SAUCE 87

DINNER 88

ONE-PAN CURRIED CHICKEN THIGHS AND CAULIFLOWER 88

SNACKS 89

SAVORY COLLARD CHIPS 89

DAY 18 90

BREAKFAST 90

BLUEBERRY-OAT PANCAKES 90

LUNCH 91

BELL PEPPER 'N GARLIC MEDLEY ON SEA BASS 91

DINNER 93

ASIAN CHICKEN SATAY 93

SNACKS 94

WALNUT BUTTER ON CRACKER 94
DAY 19 94

BREAKFAST 94

SUMMER VEGETABLE OMELET 94

LUNCH 95

MIXED GREEN LEAF AND CITRUS SALAD 95

DINNER 96

ASIAN-STYLE PAN-FRIED CHICKEN 96

SNACKS 97

ROASTED MINT CARROTS 97
DAY 20 99

BREAKFAST 99

GARDEN SALAD WITH STRAWBERRIES 99

LUNCH 100

CREAMY GORGONZOLA POLENTA WITH SUMMER SQUASH SAUTÉ 100

DINNER 101

SQUASH AND EGGPLANT CASSEROLE 101

SNACKS 103

CINNAMON APPLE CHIPS 103
DAY 21 103

BREAKFAST **103**

GREEN BREAKFAST SOUP 104

LUNCH **105**

CUCUMBER AND RADISH SALAD 105

DINNER **105**

CHICKEN, PASTA, AND BROCCOLI BAKE 105

SNACKS **107**

ROASTED BANANAS WITH CHOCOLATE YOGURT CREAM 107

CHAPTER 2: SHOPPING LIST **109**

CONCLUSION **119**

PART 2 .... **121**

THE STRUCTURE OF THE KIDNEY **122**

CHRONIC KIDNEY FAILURE 123
WHAT ARE THE CAUSES OF CHRONIC KIDNEY FAILURE? 124
WHAT SYMPTOMS CAN OCCUR? 125
MAIN CAUSES & RISK FACTORS 126

CHRONIC KIDNEY WEAKNESS: FIRST SIGNS & SYMPTOMS **129**

KIDNEY WEAKNESS (CHRONIC): EFFECTS & COMPLICATIONS 133
PREGNANCY & KIDNEY WEAKNESS 135

CHRONIC RENAL INSUFFICIENCY: TREATMENT **138**

DIET IN RENAL INSUFFICIENCY 141
CHRONIC RENAL INSUFFICIENCY 142
NON-ALLOWED FOODS 144
ALLOWED AND RECOMMENDED FOODS 146
BEHAVIORAL ADVICE 147
PRACTICAL TIPS 148
SIMPLE NUTRITION TIPS 148

DIETARY GUIDELINES **150**

CAUTION FOR "DIET SALT" OR "REPLACEMENT SALT" 155

TOP 15 KIDNEY-FRIENDLY NUTRITION FOR PEOPLE WITH KIDNEY PROBLEMS **157**

TIPS TO PREVENT KIDNEY DAMAGE 161

TIPS FOR EATING LESS SALT.. 162

TIPS FOR EATING LESS SATURATED FAT 166

TIPS AGAINST FOOD INFECTIONS 167

TIPS AGAINST CONSTIPATION 168

STOP SMOKING: 10 PITFALLS AND TIPS. **170**

90+ RECIPES **173**

CIABATTA 173

RICE WITH STIR-FRIED CHICKEN FILLET AND BOK CHOY 174

AMARANTH MUESLI BARS 175

RED CURRANT JELLY 176

RASPBERRY JELLY WITH MINT 176

BLACKBERRY AND ELDERBERRY JELLY 177

PAPAYA AND ORANGE JAM 178

CARROT DRINK... 178

SPICY APPLE AND PINEAPPLE JUICE 179

GREEN FRUIT PACKETS 179

STRAWBERRY PAPAYA DRINK 180

ORANGE BULGUR 181

ARTICHOKE CREAM ON CORN WAFFLES.. 182

OAT AND PINE NUT CRUNCHIES 182

MANGO AND RASPBERRY COCKTAIL 183

MELONS AND SPINACH JUICE 184

BAGUETTE 184

Part 1

Introduction

The guide is intended for people with chronic kidney disease, as well as for their loved ones. Also, the guide tries to answer questions about nutrition and daily lifestyle.

Key recommendations

Chronic kidney disease is a slow-moving disease and does not cause the patient a lot of complaints in the initial stages. The group of diseases of chronic kidney disease includes several kidney diseases, in which case the renal function decreases for several years or decades. If you have been diagnosed with chronic kidney disease, changes may need to be made to your lifestyle and diet to keep your kidney function at the proper level. You can do a lot to help with the treatment.

- Regularly visit the doctor and be sure to do the tests with the frequency as prescribed by the doctor. Know the value of your main indicators - glomerular filtration rate (GFR) and serum creatinine level.
- Strictly monitor the treatment plan and discuss with the doctor or nurse all questions and problems arising from the disease and its treatment.
- Use only those drugs that have been prescribed and approved by a doctor. Some medicines can damage kidneys. Know the names of their drugs and their doses. Take them only as prescribed by your doctor.
- Use only those nutritional supplements and vitamins that your doctor recommended.
- When visiting doctors, always inform them that you have chronic kidney disease. You must also inform your doctor that another doctor has prescribed a course of treatment for you.
- If you need to do examinations with a contrast agent (for example, computed tomography, angiography, magnetic

resonance imaging), then discuss them first with your doctor and follow his instructions.

- If you have high blood pressure, you should know the recommended level of blood pressure and keep it under control. It is essential to protect the kidneys.
- If you have diabetes, monitor your blood sugar levels, stick to your prescribed diet, and take medicine.
- Know your cholesterol level. When you increase your cholesterol level, carefully monitor your recommended lifestyle. To do this, it is crucial to maintain a diet, an active lifestyle, weight maintenance at a level that is normal for you, and medication.
- Observe a healthy diet. If you need to limit the intake of any product, plan the composition of your meal so that you can get from it all the necessary nutrients and calories.
- If you are overweight, try to find safe methods of losing weight with your doctor. Losing body weight will help the kidneys to work longer in normal mode.
- Do not skip meals or stay without food for several hours.
- Try to eat 4-5 small amounts of food instead of 1-2 main meals.
- Drink enough fluids. If your doctor has prescribed you limited fluid intake, then it is essential to follow this recommendation. If you are still tormented by thirst, you can quench it by putting a slice of lemon in your mouth, or rinsing your mouth with water.
- Reduce the amount of salt consumed with food.
- Be physically active. Physical activity helps to reduce blood pressure, blood sugar, and cholesterol levels, and also helps you better cope with the disease.
- If you smoke, find an opportunity to quit this habit.
- Try to be active in the process of maintaining your health.
- Search and find information about chronic kidney disease and its treatment.

- If you have diabetes, monitor your blood sugar levels, stick to your prescribed diet, and take medicine.
- Know your cholesterol level. When you increase your cholesterol level, carefully monitor your recommended lifestyle. To do this, it is very important to maintain a diet, an active lifestyle, weight maintenance at a level that is normal for you, and medication.
- Observe a healthy diet. If you need to limit the intake of any product, plan the composition of your meal so that you can get from it all the necessary nutrients and calories.
- If you are overweight, try to find safe methods of losing weight with your doctor. Losing body weight will help the kidneys to work longer in normal mode.
- Do not skip meals or stay without food for several hours.
- Try to eat 4-5 small amounts of food instead of 1-2 main meals.
- Drink enough fluids. If your doctor has prescribed you limited fluid intake, then it is essential to follow this recommendation. If you are still tormented by thirst, you can quench it by putting a slice of lemon in your mouth, or rinsing your mouth with water.
- Reduce the amount of salt consumed with food.
- Be physically active. Physical activity helps to reduce blood pressure, blood sugar, and cholesterol levels, and also helps you better cope with the disease.
- If you smoke, find an opportunity to quit this habit.
- Try to be active in the process of maintaining your health.
- Search and find information about chronic kidney disease and its treatment.

C t swarming and renal function

Usually, a person has two kidneys, which resemble beans in shape and lie adjacent to the posterior abdominal wall under the ribs. Both buds are the size of a clenched male fist.

Healthy kidneys:

Engaged in the removal from the body of end products of metabolism and excess fluid

- Help keep blood pressure under control
- Help produce red blood cells
- Help keep bones healthy

Healthy kidney

Imagine your kidneys are a coffee filter. When making coffee, the filter holds the coffee powder, but at the same time allows the liquid to move through it.

The kidneys do something similar - they retain, leave the necessary substances in the body, but at the same time filter out the substances, it does not need. The final metabolic products that filter out the kidneys appear in the body during the breakdown processes related to nutrition, drinking, medication, and normal muscular work.

There are about a million small filters in each kidney called glomeruli. Primary urine is formed in the glomeruli, which flows through the small tubules, where some of the fluid is sucked back. The functional unit of the kidney is the nephron - a specific structure consisting of the glomerulus and the tubule system. The nephrons remove residual substances and excess fluid in the form of urine into the renal pelvis, then urine is transferred to the ureters, and then into the bladder.

In the case of chronic kidney disease, renal function deteriorates the kidneys can no longer sufficiently filter residues and purify the blood. The ability of the kidneys to filter assessed based on a special indicator glomerular filtration rate (GFR).

CAUSES CHRONIC KIDNEY DISEASE

Chronic kidney disease is a slow-moving disease and does not cause the patient a lot of complaints in the initial stages. The group of diseases of chronic kidney disease includes several kidney diseases, in which case the renal function decreases for several years or decades. With the help of timely diagnosis and treatment can slow down and even stop the progression of kidney disease.

In international studies of renal function in many people, it was found that almost every tenth kidney was found to have impaired kidney function to one degree or another.

The three most common causes of chronic kidney disease are diabetes, high blood pressure, and glomerulonephritis.

- Diabetes - in the case of this disease, various organs are damaged, including the kidneys and heart, as well as blood vessels, nerves, and eyes. With long-term diabetic kidney damage, many patients increase blood pressure and need to be treated accordingly.

- High blood pressure (hypertension, primary arterial hypertension) - during hypertension, blood pressure cannot be controlled, and it begins to exceed the limits of the norm (more than 140/90 mm Hg). If this condition is permanent, it can cause chronic kidney disease, brain stroke, or myocardial infarction.

- Glomerulonephritis is a disease that occurs as a result of a breakdown in the immune system, during which the filtration function of the kidneys disrupts immune inflammation. The disease can affect only the kidneys and can spread to the entire body (vacuities, lupus nephritis). Glomerulonephritis is often accompanied by high blood pressure.

Many other conditions can cause chronic kidney disease, for example:

Hereditary diseases - such as, for example, polycystic kidney disease, due to which over the years a large number of cysts appear in the kidneys, which damage the functioning renal tissue and therefore develop renal failure. Other hereditary diseases of the kidneys are much less common (Alport syndrome, Fabry disease, etc.)

problems caused by obstructions in the kidneys and urine excretion - such as congenital malformations of the ureter, kidney stones, tumors or enlargement of the prostate gland in men repeated urinary tract infections or pyelonephritis.

Does everyone have chronic kidney disease?

Chronic kidney disease can develop at any age. The greatest risk of getting sick is in people who have one or more of the following risk factors:

- Diabetes
- High blood pressure
- Family members have previously had kidney disease
- Age over 50
- Long-term consumption of drugs that can damage the kidneys
- Overweight or obesity

What are the symptoms of chronic kidney disease?

If chronic kidney disease progresses, then the blood levels of end products of metabolism increase, this in turn, is the cause of feeling unwell. Various health problems may occur, such as high blood pressure, anemia (anemia), bone disease, premature cardiovascular calcification, discoloration, composition and volume of urine.

As the disease progresses, the main symptoms can be:

- Weakness, feeling of weakness
- Dyspnea
- Trouble sleeping
- Lack of appetite
- Dry skin, itchy skin
- Muscle cramps especially at night
- Swelling in the legs
- Swelling around the eyes, especially in the morning

Stage of Chronic Kidney Disease

There are a total of five stages of chronic kidney disease. The severity of kidney damage depends on the glomerular filtration rate (GFR), which is used to evaluate kidney function. Further treatment depends on the severity of chronic kidney disease.

Regularly visit the doctor and be sure to do the tests with the frequency as prescribed by the doctor.

Required for a wee complaints and concerns with your doctor or nurse, in no case, do not self-medicate and self-diagnosis.

Diagnose With Chronic Kidney Disease

To diagnose kidney disease, there are two simple tests that your family doctor can prescribe.

1. Blood test: glomerular filtration rate (GFR) and serum creatinine level. Creatinine is one of those end products of protein metabolism, the level of which in the blood depends on age, gender, muscle mass, nutrition, physical activity, on which foods before taking the sample (for example, a lot of meat was eaten), and some drugs. Creatinine is excreted from the body through the kidneys, and if the work of the kidneys slows down, the level of creatinine in the blood plasma increases. Determining the level of creatinine alone is not sufficient for the diagnosis of chronic kidney disease since its value begins to exceed the upper limit of the norm only when GFRdecreased by half. GFR is calculated using a formula that includes four parameters that take into account the creatinine reading, age, gender, and race of the patient. GFR shows at what level is the ability of the kidneys to filter. In the case of chronic kidney disease, the GFR indicator indicates the stage of the severity of kidney disease.

2. Urine analysis: the content of albumin in the urine is determined; also, the values of albumin and creatinine in the urine are determined by each other. Albumin is a protein in the urine that usually enters the urine in minimal quantities. Even a small increase in the level of albumin in the urine in

some people may be an early sign of incipient kidney disease, especially in those with diabetes and high blood pressure. In the case of normal kidney function, albumin in the urine should be no more than 3 mg/mmol (or 30 mg / g). If albumin excretion increases even more, then it already speaks of kidney disease. If albumin excretion exceeds 300 mg / g, other proteins are excreted into the urine, and this condition is called proteinuria.

If the kidney is healthy, then albumin does not enter the urine.

In the case of an injured kidney, albumin begins to enter the urine.

If, after receiving the results of the urine analysis, the doctor suspects that there is a kidney disease, then an additional urine analysis is performed for albumin. If albuminuria or proteinuria is detected again within three months, then this indicates chronic kidney disease.

Additional examinations

In kidney ultrasound examination: in the diagnosis of chronic kidney disease, it is an examination of the primary choice. Ultrasound examination allows to assess the shape of the kidneys, their size, location, as well as to determine possible changes in the kidney tissue and / or other abnormalities that may interfere with the normal functioning of the kidneys. Ultrasound examination of the kidneys does not require special training and has no risks for the patient.

If necessary, and if a urological disease is suspected, an ultrasound examination of the urinary tract can be prescribed (as well as a residual urine analysis), and an ultrasound examination of the prostate gland can be prescribed for men and referred to a urologist for a consultation. If necessary, and if a gynecological disease is suspected, a woman is referred for consultation to a gynecologist.

What you need to know about the examination with a contrast agent, if you have chronic kidney disease

Diagnostic examinations such as magnetic resonance imaging, computed tomography, and angiography are used to diagnose and treat various diseases and injuries. In many cases, intravenous and intra-arterial contrast agents (containing iodine or gadolinium) are used, which makes it possible to see the organs or blood vessels under study.

What is particularly important to do before the survey pole to gain in contrast substance?

If you are scheduled for an examination with a contrast agent, then you need to determine your GFR.

Together with your doctor, you can discuss and evaluate the benefits or harm to your health. If the survey is still necessary, follow the following preparation rules:

- The day before the survey and the day after the survey, drink plenty of fluids (water, tea, etc.). If you are on treatment in a hospital, then you will be injected with the necessary amount of fluid through a vein by infusion. When staying in hospital treatment after examination with a contrast agent (within 48-96 hours), it is usually prescribed to determine the level of creatinine in the blood to assess renal function. In the outpatient examination with a contrast agent, your family doctor will be able to evaluate your kidney function.
- Discuss with your doctor the questions about which medications should not be taken before the examination with a contrast agent. Some drugs (antibiotics, drugs against high blood pressure, etc.) along with contrasting substances begin to act as a poison. The day before and the day after the examination, in no case should you take metformin - a cure for diabetes.
- Between the two examinations with a contrast agent, at the first opportunity, sufficient time should be left for the contrast agent that was used during the first examination to leave the body. It is important to exclude repeated examinations with a large amount of contrast material.

Effect Of A Contrast Agent On The Kidneys

Sometimes a contrast agent can damage the kidneys. The greatest risk is kidney damage in patients with chronic kidney disease. There are two rare, but very serious diseases that can occur as a result of the administration of a contrast agent: nephropathy and nephrogenic systemic fibrosis.

What is nephropathy resulting from the administration of a contrast agent?

Nephropathy resulting from the administration of a contrast agent is rare; it can occur in about 6% of patients. The risk of getting sick is especially high in diabetics, as well as in people with chronic kidney disease.

In the case of nephropathy caused by a contrast agent, there is a sharp decrease in renal function within 48-72 hours after the examination. In most cases, this condition disappears, and the person recovers, but in rare cases, serious problems can occur both in the kidneys and in the cardiovascular system.

Nephrogenic Systemic Fibrosis

It is a very rare but serious illness that damages the skin and other organs. The disease can develop over 24 hours to 3 months from the day of the treatment with a contrast agent that includes gadolinium.

This disease is very rare, and in people with mild renal dysfunction or normal kidney function, the occurrence of nephrogenic systemic fibrosis was not observed.

- Know the value of your main indicators - glomerular filtration rate (GFR) and serum creatinine level. Ask your doctor to explain their meaning.
- E If you n have zhno do surveys with contrast medium (e.g., computed tomography, angiography, magnetic resonance imaging), discuss it first of all with your doctor and follow his instructions.

What are the treatment options for chronic kidney disease?

The possibilities of treating chronic kidney disease depend on the stage of the severity of the kidney disease, on concomitant diseases and other health problems.

Treatment may include:

- Treatment of high blood pressure
- Diabetes treatment
- In the case of excess weight - its reduction

Lifestyle changes: healthy eating, reduced salt intake, adequate physical activity, stopping smoking, limiting alcohol intake.

Dialysis treatment and kidney transplantation in the case of chronic kidney disease in the latter stages of developmental severity (stage 5).

Psychological consultation and support.

Treatment of high blood pressure in case of chronic kidney disease

What is blood pressure?

Blood pressure is the pressure that is created by the blood flowing through the blood vessels to the walls of the blood vessels. The unit for measuring blood pressure is a millimeter of mercury (abbreviated mm of mercury), and two numbers determine blood pressure — systolic and diastolic blood pressure — for example, 130/80 mm of mercury. Art. Systolic pressure or upper-pressure value means the level of blood pressure at the moment when the heart releases blood from the chamber, i.e., while compressing the heart.

Diastolic pressure or lower pressure value means the level of blood pressure at the moment when the heart is at the moment of   relaxation.
High blood pressure (hypertension) is a common disease, and often the person himself does not know that his indicator of pressure is above normal. As the disease progresses, the main symptoms may include:

- Headache
- Rapid Heartbeat
- Fatigue
- Imbalance

Untreated, elevated pressure can cause kidney damage, cardiovascular diseases, stroke, or eye diseases. High blood pressure can cause damage to the renal arteries and reduce the functional ability of the kidneys. The kidneys with damaged arteries can no longer excrete end products of metabolism or excess fluid from the body. Due to excess fluid, the pressure starts to rise even more.

It is essential to keep blood pressure within normal limits. Regardless of age, blood pressure should not exceed 140/90 mmHg.

If you have chronic kidney disease and there are additional risk factors (for example, albuminuria, diabetes, diseases of the cardiovascular system), the blood pressure should be kept at 130 / 80 mm Hg.

The best way to measure blood pressure and to keep it under control is to measure your blood pressure at home (and in a pharmacy) with a blood pressure monitor.

Discuss your treatment plan with your doctor. If necessary, the doctor will refer you to a cardiologist or an eye doctor for control tests. In addition to taking medicine in the form of pills and controlling blood pressure, a healthy lifestyle plays an important role in the treatment (see. How can you help the treatment yourself?).

COOKING TIPS

Hopefully, by now, you know more about the symptoms, causes, and stages of kidney disease. You also know a little more about kidney-friendly foods as well as foods you should potentially limit or avoid. This chapter outlines the best cooking methods for a healthy diet, which is in line with healthy eating advice in general. It also provides ways of combating sodium and potassium.

COMBATING SODIUM:

Salt is often overused to season our foods and act as preservatives in packaged foods. In fact, taste tests show that as little as one-eighth of a teaspoon is enough for most people to notice. Reduce the amount of salt you add to foods gradually and always check the labels of ingredients for their sodium levels.

If using canned vegetables, ensure the juice or broth has no added salt by checking the labels; fresh vegetables are always a better option. You can easily make broths and soups out of leftover vegetables or bones from chicken, turkey and even beef. A chicken stock recipe is included in the poultry section. Herbs and spices, as well as balsamic or white vinegar, can be used to replace salt when cooking or dressing foods. Sometimes, something sweet can be used for a surprising twist on your favorite meal, for example, a squeeze of fresh lime or lemon juice. Likewise, different cooking methods result in a variety of flavors from the same ingredients! Experiment with baking and roasting as well as grilling to liven up the same foods in the kitchen..

COMBATING POTASSIUM:

Boiling vegetables helps reduce potassium; if you've got extra time or you're really prepared, soaking them in warm water for a few hours helps this process. Cleaning and peeling potatoes and boiling twice is sufficient enough for stripping excess potassium out of the potatoes. When making stews and soups it is better to boil the vegetables first so as not to allow potassium to soak into the rest of the pot. If cooking with frozen or canned vegetables, they should be rinsed and soaked prior to use in order to reduce potassium levels. Low-sodium labelled products are not the ideal choice as these often contain other chemicals that are harmful to the body. Instead, use the methods described above to reduce potassium as much as possible and try using ingredients with a low potassium content where you can.

CONSIDER YOUR LIFESTYLE

Follows the tips below to make the transition to a healthy, kidney friendly diet as easy as possible.

- Eat a large breakfast, a medium-sized lunch, and a small dinner.
- Increase consumption of vegetables and fruits daily.
- Switch to olive oil based dressings.
- Try healthy snacks instead of quick and processed snacks e.g. roasted kale chips, plain yogurt, fruits and nuts in moderation.
- Eating smaller meals with a healthy snack in between will work for those needing to control calorie intake as well as those who have lost their appetite.
- Stay away from juices and sodas as they both contain high amounts of processed ingredients and sugar.
- Drink fresh water and green teas, but be aware of how much liquid you should be consuming each day.
- Don't eat after 8 pm to allow your body and kidneys time to function before sleep.
- Find an activity or hobby to prevent boredom eating.
- Get into the habit of reading labels on foods and looking for sodium, potassium, phosphorous, protein and calorie amounts.
- Eat a balanced diet to include protein, healthy fats and carbohydrates according to your diagnosis and personal needs.
- Stop smoking.

- Stay positive by asking friends and family members to try the healthy eating with you.

- If you have a bad day, don't let it throw you off for good.

- Log your symptoms as well as what you eat in a journal every day. This will help you keep track not only of how much and what types of foods you've eaten but also how they make you feel.

- Keep up with scheduled appointments and monitor your blood pressure to ensure it is not too high.

- If you're diabetic, ensure you monitor your condition and consult your doctor about specific sugar recommendations.

- Seek professional advice early as well as the support from loved ones. This can be an incredibly emotional time and you shouldn't have to experience it alone. Therapy might even be an option if you wish to talk about your feelings to a third party.

EXERCISE

The level of exercise you can safely perform while dealing with your chronic kidney disease will vary greatly depending on your current prognosis, the symptoms you are showing and your general level of physical fitness. Exercise is known to be especially helpful in the early stages of the disease and can help to fight off the initial feelings of fatigue that many people experience.

Exercise is useful for those who are looking to lose weight as a way to help mitigate numerous conditions that can lead to chronic kidney failure. Exercise can also strengthen the heart and is also known to help with anxiety as well as depression.

For those who have to limit their fluid intake, strenuous exercise is not advised as you will become dehydrated and need to consume higher quantities of water. In this case yoga and light walks are advised to keep fit and healthy whilst not exerting yourself too much. Speak with your healthcare professional for specific guidance.

Chapter 1: THE 21 DAYS MEAL PLAN
Day 1

Breakfast Recipe
Quesadillas with Pears

Stage 1: Slight kidney damage, and usually no symptoms. (eGFR > 90 mL)

Ingredients:

- 2 tbsps minced onion (green, red, or yellow)
- ½ cup finely chopped green or red peppers
- 1 cup pear cubes (fresh or canned/drained)
- 1 cup grated cheese (try cheddar or jack)
- 4 medium whole wheat tortillas

Directions:

1. On a clean cutting board, lay two tortillas. You may also use two plates depending on your preference. In each tortilla, place or spread ¼ cheese then divide the onions, peppers, and pears between the two tortillas.
2. Spread the remaining cheese onto the 2 tortillas then top off with the remaining two other tortillas. Medium-heat a pan then cook for 2 to 4 minutes the first quesadilla.
3. Once the bottom begins to turn brown, gently turn it to cook the other side until it turns brown, too. Slide onto plate then cook the other or second quesadilla. Once all quesadillas are cooked, cut each into 4 pieces and they are ready to serve.

Serves: 4   Prep Time: 10 mins.   Cook Time: 20 mins.

Calories: 302; Carbs: 33g; Protein: 13g; Fat: 15g; Phosphorus: 296mg; Potassium: 197mg; Sodium: 412mg

Lunch Recipe

Chicken and Sweet Potato Stir Fry

Stage 1: Slight kidney damage, and usually no symptoms. (eGFR > 90 mL)

Ingredients:

- ¼ tsp natural sea salt
- ½ cups quinoa, rinsed and drained
- 1 clove garlic, minced
- 1 cup frozen peas
- 1 cup water
- 1 jalapeno chili pepper, chopped
- 1 medium onion, chopped
- 1 medium-sized red bell pepper, chopped
- 1 tsp cumin, ground
- 1/8 tsp black pepper
- 12oz boneless chicken
- 1med sweet potatoes, cubed
- 3 tbsp fresh cilantro, chopped
- 4 tsp canola oil

Directions:

1. Bring to a boil water and quinoa over medium heat. Simmer until the quinoa has absorbed the water. In a small saucepan, put the sweet potatoes and enough water to cover the potatoes. Bring to a boil. Drain the potatoes and discard the water.
2. In a skillet, add the chicken and cook until brown. Transfer to a bowl. Using the same skillet, heat 2 tablespoon of oil and sauté the onions and jalapeno pepper for one minute.
3. Add the bell pepper, cumin and garlic. Cook for three minutes until the vegetables have softened. Add the peas

and chicken. Cook for two minutes before adding the sweet potato and quinoa. Stir cilantro and add salt and pepper to taste. Serve and enjoy.

Serves: 3   Prep Time: 1 min.   Cook Time: 40 mins.

Calories: 415; Carbs: 39g; Protein: 28g; Fat: 18g; Phosphorus: 410mg; Potassium: 1201mg; Sodium: 297mg

Dinner

Sea Bass with Basil-Tomato Topping

Stage 1: Slight kidney damage, and usually no symptoms. (eGFR > 90 mL)

Ingredients:

- 1 shallot, thinly sliced
- 1 tablespoon olive oil
- 1 tbsp balsamic vinegar
- Basil, 1/4 cup, chopped
- 2 cups cherry tomatoes (about 12 ounces)
- 2 garlic cloves, chopped
- 24-ounce fillets sea bass or other white fish
- 1 tsp freshly ground pepper

Directions:

1. Place a rack in upper third of oven and preheat broiler. 1) Set your broiler on to preheat. Combine oil, balsamic, tomatoes, garlic and shallot, and oil in a medium bowl, season with pepper, and toss well. Set aside.
2. Place fish in a 13x9-inch glass baking dish. Pour your mixture on top of your fish then broil until opaque.

Serves: 4   Prep Time: 10 mins.   Cook Time: 13 mins.

Calories: 245; Carbs: 13g; Protein: 33g; Fat: 7g; Phosphorus: 346mg; Potassium: 570mg; Sodium: 126mg

Snacks

Chocolate Beet Cake

Stage 1: Slight kidney damage, and usually no symptoms. (eGFR > 90 mL)

Ingredients:

- 1 cup sugar
- 2 cups all-purpose flour
- 2 teaspoons Phosphorus-Free Baking Powder
- 4 ounces unsweetened chocolate
- 4 large eggs
- ¼ cup canola oil
- 3 cups grated beets

Directions:

1. Preheat the oven to 325°F. Grease two 8-inch cake pans. In a large bowl, whisk the sugar, flour, and baking powder together. Set aside. Finely chop the chocolate, and melt in a double boiler. Let cool, and mix together with the eggs and oil. Add the wet ingredients to the dry, mixing well to blend.
2. Fold in the beets, and pour the batter into the cake pans. Cook for 40 minutes

Serves: 12   Prep Time: 10 mins.   Cook Time: 50 mins.

Calories: 270; Fat: 12g; Carbs: 39g; Protein: 6g; Phosphorus: 111mg; Potassium: 299mg; Sodium: 109mg

Day 2

Breakfast

Open-Faced Bagel Breakfast Sandwich

Stage 1: Slight kidney damage, and usually no symptoms. (eGFR > 90 mL)

Ingredients:

- 1 multigrain bagel, halved
- 2 tablespoons cream cheese, divided
- 2 slices tomato
- 1 slice red onion
- Freshly ground black pepper
- 1 cup microgreens

Directions:

1. In a toaster or oven, lightly toast the bagel. Spread 1 tablespoon of cream cheese on each of the bagel halves, and top each half with 1 slice of tomato and a couple rings of onion. Season with the black pepper. Top each half with ½ cup of microgreens and serve.

Serves: 2   Prep Time: 5 mins.   Cook Time: 5 mins.

Calories: 456; Fat: 6g; Protein: 5g; Protein: 5g; Phosphorus: 98mg; Potassium: 163mg; Sodium: 195mg

Lunch

Swordfish and Citrus Salsa Delight

Stage 1: Slight kidney damage, and usually no symptoms. (eGFR > 90 mL)

Ingredients:

- 1 ½ pounds swordfish steaks
- 1 tbsp pineapple juice concentrate (thawed)
- ¼ tsp cayenne pepper
- 1 tbsp olive oil
- ½ cup fresh orange juice
- 1 tbsp chopped fresh cilantro
- 2 tsp. white sugar
- 1 tbsp diced red bell pepper
- 3 tbsp. orange juice
- 2 jalapeno peppers (seeded and minced)
- ¼ cup diced fresh mango
- **Pineapple, ½ cup,** canned, chunks (**with juice**)
- 1 orange (peeled, seeded, and cubed)

Directions:

1. In a bowl, make the salsa by combining and mixing well the cilantro, oranges, sugar, pineapple chunks, diced red bell pepper, minced jalapenos, mango, and 3 tablespoons orange juice. Cover the bowl and refrigerate.
2. Mix the pineapple juice concentrate, cayenne pepper, olive oil and ½ cup orange juice in a non-reactive bowl. Add swordfish steaks in the bowl of pineapple juice mixture. Coat and turn well. Ensure to marinate for about 30 minutes. On a gas grill, set heat to medium-high. For 12 to 15 minutes in total, grill the swordfish then serve with salsa.

Serves: 6   Prep Time: 10 mins.   Cook Time: 30 mins.

Calories: 404; Carbs: 13g; Protein: 30g; Fat: 23g; Phosphorus: 251mg; Potassium: 486mg; Sodium: 68mg

Dinner

Aromatic Chicken and Cabbage Stir-Fry

Stage 1: Slight kidney damage, and usually no symptoms. (eGFR > 90 mL)

Ingredients:

- 1 teaspoon canola oil
- 10 ounces boneless, skinless chicken breast, thinly sliced
- 3 cups green cabbage, thinly sliced
- 1 tablespoon cornstarch
- 1 teaspoon ground ginger
- ½ teaspoon garlic powder
- ¼ cup water
- Freshly ground black pepper

Directions:

1. Set your oil in a skillet over medium heat to get hot. Add the chicken and cook, stirring often, until browned and cooked through. Add the cabbage to the pan, and cook for another 2 to 3 minutes, until the cabbage is tender but still crisp and green.
2. In a small bowl, mix the cornstarch, ginger, garlic, and water. Add the mixture to the pan, and continue cooking until the sauce has slightly thickened, about 1 minute. Season with pepper.

Serves: 4   Prep Time: 10 mins.   Cook Time: 10 mins.

Calories: 396; Fat: 2g; Carbs: 5g; Protein: 15g; Phosphorus: 15mg; Potassium: 140mg; Sodium: 156mg

Snacks

Vegetable Lentil Soup

Stage 1: Slight kidney damage, and usually no symptoms. (eGFR > 90 mL)

Ingredients:

- 1 tablespoon extra-virgin olive oil
- ½ sweet onion, diced
- 2 carrots, diced
- 2 celery stalks, diced
- ½ cup lentils
- 5 cups Simple Chicken Broth or low-sodium store-bought chicken stock
- 2 cups sliced chard leaves
- Freshly ground black pepper
- Juice of 1 lemon

Directions:

1. In a medium stockpot over medium-high heat, heat the olive oil. Add the onion and stir until softened, about 3 to 5 minutes. Add the carrots, celery, lentils, and broth.
2. Bring to a boil, reduce the heat and simmer, uncovered, for 15 minutes, until the lentils are tender. Add the chard and cook for 3 additional minutes, until wilted. Season with the pepper and lemon juice. Serve.

Serves: 4   Prep Time: 10 mins.   Cook Time: 25 mins.

Calories: 695; Fat: 6g; Carbs: 25g; Protein: 13g; Phosphorus: 228mg; Potassium: 707mg; Sodium: 157mg

Day 3

Breakfast

Peach Berry Parfait

Stage 1: Slight kidney damage, and usually no symptoms. (eGFR > 90 mL)

Ingredients:

- 1 cup plain, unsweetened yogurt, divided
- 1 teaspoon vanilla extract
- 1 small peach, diced
- ½ cup blueberries
- 2 tablespoons walnut pieces

Directions:

1. In a small bowl, mix together the yogurt and vanilla. Add 2 tablespoons of yogurt to each of 2 cups. Divide the diced peach and the blueberries between the cups, and top with the remaining yogurt. Sprinkle each cup with 1 tablespoon of walnut pieces.

Serves: 2   Prep Time: 5 mins.   Cook Time: 0 mins.

Calories: 591; Fat:10g; Carbs: 14g; Fiber: 14g; Protein: 12g; Phosphorus: 189mg; Potassium: 327mg; Sodium: 40mg

Lunch

Red Coleslaw with Apple

Stage 1: Slight kidney damage, and usually no symptoms. (eGFR > 90 mL)

Ingredients:

- 3 cups shredded red cabbage
- ½ cup shredded carrots
- ¼ cup finely chopped scallions
- Juice of 2 lemons
- 1 tablespoon honey
- 1 tablespoon extra-virgin olive oil
- 1 large tart apple, peeled and finely diced
- Freshly ground black pepper

Directions:

1. In a large bowl, add the cabbage, carrots, scallions, lemon juice, honey, olive oil, and apple. Mix well and refrigerate for 30 minutes to chill. Toss with black pepper right before serving.

Serves: 4   Prep Time: 10 mins.   Cook Time: 0 mins.

Calories: 494; Fat: 4g; Carbs: 16g; Fiber: 3g; Protein: 2g; Phosphorus: 28mg; Potassium: 303mg; Sodium: 281mg

Dinner

Chicken Soup with Kale and Sweet Potatoes

Stage 1: Slight kidney damage, and usually no symptoms. (eGFR > 90 mL)

Ingredients:

- 1-inch thumb sized Fresh ginger, peeled and grated
- Pepper to taste
- 3 cups water
- 3 cups low-sodium chicken broth
- 2 tbsp. apple cider vinegar
- 10 grape tomatoes, halved
- 3 cups kale, roughly chopped
- 1 lb. sweet potatoes, peeled and chopped
- 3 celery stalks, chopped
- 4 cloves garlic, diced
- 1 medium-sized onion
- 2 ½ tbsp. olive oil
- 1 lb. skinless, boneless chicken breasts

Directions:

1. With pepper, season chicken to taste. On medium high fire, place soup pot and add oil. Pan fry chicken until golden brown, around 4 minutes per side. Remove chicken from pot and put aside for the meantime.
2. In same pot, add onion, garlic and celery. Sauté for 7-8 minutes or until tender. Pour vinegar and sauté for a minute. Add water, chicken broth, tomatoes, kale, and sweet potatoes and bring to a boil. Once boiling, slow fire to a simmer and cook for 20 minutes.
3. While waiting, tear chicken for a pulled effect, with hands. Fifteen minutes into simmering time, add chicken to soup to heat through. To serve, spoon soup into bowls and top with freshly grated ginger.

Serves: 6   Prep Time: 15 mins.   Cook Time: 1 hr.

Calories: 472; Carbs: 20g; Protein: 28g; Fat: 10g; Phosphorus: 280mg; Potassium: 884mg; Sodium: 429mg

Snacks

Herbed Cabbage Stew

Stage 1: Slight kidney damage, and usually no symptoms. (eGFR > 90 mL)

Ingredients:

- 1 teaspoon unsalted butter
- ½ large sweet onion, chopped
- 1 teaspoon minced garlic
- 6 cups shredded green cabbage
- 3 celery stalks, chopped with the leafy tops
- 1 scallion, both green and white parts, chopped
- 2 tablespoons chopped fresh parsley
- 2 tablespoons freshly squeezed lemon juice
- 1 tablespoon chopped fresh thyme
- 1 teaspoon chopped savory
- 1 teaspoon chopped fresh oregano
- Water
- green beans, 1 cup, chopped
- Freshly ground black pepper

Directions:

1. In a medium stockpot over medium-high heat, melt the butter. Sauté the onion and garlic in the melted butter for about 3 minutes or until the vegetables are softened. Add the cabbage, celery, scallion, parsley, lemon juice, thyme, savory, and oregano to the pot, and add enough water to cover the vegetables by about 4 inches.
2. Bring the soup to a boil, reduce the heat to low, and simmer the soup for about 25 minutes or until the vegetables are

tender. Add the green beans and simmer 3 minutes. Season with pepper.

Serves: 6   Prep Time: 20 mins.   Cook Time: 35 mins.
Calories: 533; Fat: 1g; Carbs: 6g; Phosphorus: 29mg; Potassium: 187mg; Sodium: 20mg; Protein: 1g

Day 4

Breakfast

Egg in The Hole

Stage 2: Mild damage in kidneys (eGFR = 60–89 mL)

Ingredients:
- 2 (½-inch-thick) slices Italian bread
- ¼ cup unsalted butter
- 2 eggs
- 2 tablespoons chopped fresh chives
- Pinch cayenne pepper
- Freshly ground black pepper

Directions:
1. Using a cookie cutter or a small glass, cut a 2-inch round from the center of each piece of bread. Set your butter to melt in a large skillet over medium-high heat, melt the butter. Place the bread in the skillet, toast it for 1 minute, and then flip the bread over.
2. Crack the eggs into the holes the center of the bread and cook for about 2 minutes or until the eggs are set and the bread is golden brown. Top with chopped chives, cayenne pepper, and black pepper.
3. Cook the bread for another 2 minutes. Transfer an egg-in-the-hole to each plate to serve.

Calories: 304; Fat: 29g; Carbs: 12g; Phosphorus: 119mg; Potassium: 109mg; Sodium: 204mg; Protein: 9g

Lunch

Lemon-Herb Chicken

Stage 2: Mild damage in kidneys (eGFR = 60–89 mL)

Ingredients:

- 12 ounces boneless, skinless chicken breast, cut into 8 strips
- 1 small egg white
- 2 tablespoons water, divided
- ½ cup breadcrumbs
- ¼ cup unsalted butter, divided
- Juice of 1 lemon
- Zest of 1 lemon
- 1 tablespoon fresh chopped basil
- 1 teaspoon fresh chopped thyme
- Lemon slices, for garnish

Directions:

1. Place the chicken strips between 2 sheets of plastic wrap and pound each flat with a mallet or rolling pin. In a medium bowl, whisk together the egg and 1 tablespoon water.
2. Put the breadcrumbs in another medium bowl. Dredge the chicken strips, one at a time, in the egg, then the breadcrumbs, and set the breaded strips aside on a plate. Set 2 tbsp of your butter to melt in a skillet on medium heat.
3. Cook the strips in the butter for about 3 minutes, turning once, or until they are golden and cooked through. Transfer the chicken to a plate. Add the lemon juice, lemon zest, basil,

thyme, and remaining 1 tablespoon water to the skillet and stir until the mixture simmers.
4. Remove the sauce from the heat and stir in the remaining 2 tablespoons butter. Serve the chicken with the lemon sauce drizzled over the top and garnished with lemon slices.
5.

Serves: 4   Prep Time: 20 mins.   Cook Time: 15 mins.

Calories: 455; Fat: 14g; Carbs: 11g; Phosphorus: 180mg; Potassium: 321mg; Sodium: 261mg; Protein: 20g

Dinner

Chicken Chow Mein

Stage 2: Mild damage in kidneys (eGFR = 60–89 mL)

Ingredients:

- 2 teaspoons cornstarch
- 1 tablespoon water
- 1 teaspoon low-sodium soy sauce
- 1 teaspoon rice wine
- 1 teaspoon sugar
- 1 teaspoon sesame oil
- 2 teaspoons canola oil
- 3 garlic cloves, minced
- 8 ounces boneless, skinless chicken thighs, thinly sliced
- 2 cups shredded green cabbage
- 1 carrot, julienned
- 4 scallions, cut into 2-inch pieces
- 10 ounces chow mein noodles, cooked according to package directions

- 1 cup mung bean sprouts

Directions:

1. In a small bowl, mix the cornstarch, water, and soy sauce. Stir in the rice wine, sugar, and sesame oil, mixing well. Set aside. In a large skillet or wok over medium-high heat, heat the canola oil.
2. Add the garlic, and cook until just fragrant, stirring constantly. Add the chicken, and cook for 1 minute, stirring, until the chicken is browned but not cooked through.
3. Add the cabbage, carrot, and scallions, and cook for 1 to 2 minutes, until the cabbage begins to wilt, and the chicken is cooked through. Add the noodles and toss with the chicken and vegetables. Pour in the sauce and stir to coat. Add the bean sprouts and stir. Remove from the heat and serve.

Serves: 6   Prep Time: 10 mins.   Cook Time: 15 mins.

Calories: 542; Fat: 18g; Carbs: 34g; Protein: 13g; Phosphorus: 169mg; Potassium: 308mg; Sodium: 289mg

Snacks

Chicken Pho

Stage 2: Mild damage in kidneys (eGFR = 60–89 mL)

Ingredients:

- 5 cups Simple Chicken Broth or low-sodium store-bought chicken stock
- 1-inch piece ginger, cut lengthwise into 2 or 3 strips
- 1 cup cooked chicken breast, diced
- Several fresh Thai basil sprigs
- 1 cup mung bean sprouts

- 1 lime, cut into wedges
- 1 jalapeño pepper, stemmed, seeded, and thinly sliced
- 1 (16-ounce) package dried rice vermicelli noodles, cooked according to package
- 4 tablespoons (¼ cup) sliced scallions
- 4 tablespoons (¼ cup) chopped cilantro leaves

Directions:

1. In a medium stockpot over medium-high heat, add the broth and ginger, and bring to a simmer. Add the chicken and simmer for 5 minutes. Remove the ginger from the pot and discard.
2. On a plate, arrange the Thai basil, bean sprouts, lime wedges, and jalapeño slices. Distribute the noodles among four bowls. Add 1¼ cups of broth to each bowl. Top with 1 tablespoon each of the scallions and cilantro. Serve immediately, alongside the plate of garnishes.

Serves: 4   Prep Time: 10 mins.   Cook Time: 15 mins.

Calories: 525; Fat: 3g; Carbs: 55g; Protein: 21g; Phosphorus: 205mg; Potassium: 389mg; Sodium: 313mg

Day 5

Breakfast

Broccoli Basil Quiche

Stage 2: Mild damage in kidneys (eGFR = 60–89 mL)

Ingredients:

- 1 store-bought frozen piecrust
- 2 cups finely chopped broccoli
- 1 tomato, chopped
- 2 scallions, chopped
- 3 eggs, beaten
- 2 tablespoons chopped basil

- 1 cup Homemade Rice Milk or unsweetened store-bought rice milk
- ½ cup crumbled feta cheese
- 1 garlic clove, minced
- 1 tablespoon all-purpose flour
- Freshly ground black pepper

Directions:

1. Preheat the oven to 425°F. Line a pie pan with the piecrust and use a fork to pierce the crust in several places. Bake the crust for 10 minutes. Remove from the oven and reduce the temperature to 325°F.
2. In a medium bowl, mix the broccoli, tomato, scallions, eggs, basil, rice milk, feta, garlic, and flour. Season with pepper. Pour the broccoli-and-egg mixture into the prepared pie pan. Bake until done (about 45 minutes). Cool slightly and serve.

Serves: 8   Prep Time: 10 mins.   Cook Time: 55 mins.

Calories: 560; Total Fat: 10g; Carbohydrates: 13g; Fiber: 1g; Protein: 6g; Phosphorus: 101mg; Potassium: 173mg; Sodium: 259mg

Lunch

Herb-Garlic Sauce over Pan Fried Fish

Stage 2: Mild damage in kidneys (eGFR = 60–89 mL)

Ingredients:

- 1 tablespoon extra-virgin olive oil
- 1 tablespoon fresh parsley roughly chopped
- 1.5 lbs. sea bass such as barramundi
- 1/2 cup low sodium chicken broth

- 1/2 teaspoon black pepper plus more if needed
- 1/4 cup all-purpose flour
- 1 tablespoon fresh oregano roughly chopped
- white wine, 1/4 cup, dry
- 2 cloves garlic minced
- 3 tablespoons butter divided
- juice of one lemon about 2 tablespoons
- 1 tablespoon fresh thyme roughly chopped

Directions:

1. Dry fish. In a shallow dish, mix together the flour and black pepper. In a large skillet, preferably nonstick, melt 1 tablespoon of the butter over medium high heat and add the olive oil.
2. Cook the fish in the skillet for 3-4 minutes on each side, until golden brown and fully cooked. Remove fish from the skillet to a plate. Add another tablespoon of butter to melt. Add garlic and cook, while stirring, until fragrant.
3. Ensure that the white wine is added to the skillet in order to deglaze any browned bits. When wine has reduced by about half, add the chicken broth and bring to a simmer. Turn off heat and stir in remaining 1 tablespoon butter, lemon juice, oregano, thyme, and parsley. Taste and adjust seasoning if necessary. Serve sauce on top of fish.

Serves: 4   Prep Time: 15 mins.   Cook Time: 10 mins.

Calories: 703; Carbs: 10g; Protein: 41g; Fat: 21g; Phosphorus: 431mg; Potassium: 628mg; Sodium: 784mg

Dinner

Parsnip and Pear Soup

Stage 2: Mild damage in kidneys (eGFR = 60–89 mL)

Ingredients:

- 1 tbsp olive oil
- Pepper to taste
- ½ tsp rosemary
- 1 tsp thyme
- 1 tsp sage
- 1 clove garlic crushed
- 1 bay leaf
- 2 pears, peeled and chopped
- 2-3 cups vegetable stock
- 2 parsnips, peeled and chopped
- 2 cups cauliflower florets
- ½ leek, washed and sliced
- 1 tbsp chives

Directions:

1. On medium fire, place a soup pot and heat oil. Once oil is hot, sauté leeks for 5 minutes. Add stock, bay leaf, herbs, pear, garlic, parsnips and cauliflower. Bring to a simmer and slow fire to medium low and continue cooking for 25 minutes.
2. With an immersion blender, puree soup until smooth. Add pepper to taste. Serve topped with chives

Serves: 4   Prep Time: 15 mins.   Cook Time: 35 mins.

Calories: 598; Carbs: 35g; Protein: 6g; Fat: 6g; Phosphorus: 146mg; Potassium: 856mg; Sodium: 381mg

Snacks

Roasted Root Vegetables

Stage 2: Mild damage in kidneys (eGFR = 60–89 mL)

Ingredients:

- 1 cup chopped turnips
- 1 cup chopped rutabaga
- 1 cup chopped parsnips
- 1 tablespoon extra-virgin olive oil
- 1 teaspoon fresh chopped rosemary
- Freshly ground black pepper

Directions:

1. Preheat the oven to 400°F. In a large bowl, toss the turnips, rutabaga, and parsnips with the olive oil and rosemary. Arrange in a single layer on a baking sheet, and season with pepper. Bake until the vegetables are tender and browned, 20 to 25 minutes, stirring once.

Serves: 6   Prep Time: 10 mins.   Cook Time: 25 mins.

Calories: 452; Fat: 2g; Carbs: 7g; Protein: 1g; Phosphorus: 35mg; Potassium: 205mg; Sodium: 22mg

Day 6
Breakfast

Herbed and Spiced Grilled Eggplant
Stage 2: Mild damage in kidneys (eGFR = 60–89 mL)

Ingredients:

- 1 tbsp chopped fresh cilantro
- ¼ tsp freshly ground black pepper
- ¼ tsp natural sea salt

- 1 tsp red wine vinegar
- 1 garlic clove, minced
- 1 tbsp light molasses
- 2 cups cherry tomatoes, halved
- ½ yellow onion, finely chopped
- 1 tbsp olive oil
- Pinch of ground cloves
- Pinch of ground nutmeg
- Pinch of ground ginger
- ½ tsp curry powder
- ½ tsp ground coriander
- ½ tsp ground cumin
- 1 tsp mustard seed
- 1 large aubergine eggplant, around 1 ½ lbs.

Directions:

1. Grease grill grate with cooking spray and preheat grill to high heat. Trim eggplant and slice in ¼-inch think lengthwise strips. Grill strips of eggplant for 5 minutes per side or until browned and tender.
2. Remove eggplants from fire and keep warm. In a small bowl, mix cloves, nutmeg, ginger, curry, coriander, cumin and mustard seed. On medium high fire, place a medium nonstick skillet and heat oil.
3. Sauté spice mixture for 30 seconds and add onions. Sauté onions for 4 minutes or until soft and translucent. Add vinegar, garlic, molasses and tomatoes. Sauté for 4 minutes or until thickened.
4. Season with pepper and salt. Turn off fire. On four plates, evenly divide grilled eggplant. Evenly top each plate of eggplant with herbed and spiced sauce. Serve and enjoy while warm.

Serves: 4   Prep Time: 15 mins.   Cook Time: 40 mins.

Calories per Serving: 537; Carbs: 23g; Protein: 3g; Fat: 6g; Phosphorus: 52mg; Potassium: 484mg; Sodium: 160mg

Lunch

Roasted Cauliflower with Mixed Greens Salad

Stage 2: Mild damage in kidneys (eGFR = 60–89 mL)

Ingredients:

- 1 small head cauliflower, cut into small florets
- 2 tablespoons extra-virgin olive oil, divided
- Freshly ground black pepper
- 6 ounces mixed baby salad greens
- 2 tablespoons walnut pieces
- 1 tablespoon apple cider vinegar

Directions:

1. Set your oven to preheat to 400°F. Toss your cauliflower with 1 tablespoon of olive oil. Season with pepper. Set to bake on a large baking sheet in a single layer.
2. Cook for 30 to 35 minutes, stirring once or twice, until tender and golden brown. Let cool for about 10 minutes. Meanwhile, mix the remaining tablespoon of olive oil and the vinegar.
3. In a large bowl, toss the mixed salad greens, walnuts, and cauliflower. Just before serving, stir in the olive-oil-and-vinegar mixture, and season with pepper.

Serves: 4   Prep Time: 10 mins.   Cook Time: 35 mins.

Calories: 408; Fat: 9g; Carbs: 5g; Fiber: 2g; Protein: 2g; Phosphorus: 42mg; Potassium: 217mg; Sodium: 50mg

Dinner

Persian Chicken

Stage 2: Mild damage in kidneys (eGFR = 60–89 mL)

Ingredients:

- ½ small sweet onion, chopped
- ¼ cup freshly squeezed lemon juice
- 1 tablespoon dried oregano
- 1 teaspoon minced garlic
- 1 teaspoon sweet paprika
- ½ teaspoon ground cumin
- ½ cup olive oil
- 5 boneless, skinless chicken thighs

Directions:

1. Put the onion, lemon juice, oregano, garlic, paprika, and cumin in a blender or food processor. Pulse a few times to mix the ingredients. With the motor running, add the olive oil until the mixture is smooth.
2. Place the chicken thighs in a large sealable freezer bag and pour the marinade into the bag. Seal the bag and place it in the refrigerator, turning the bag twice, for 2 hours.
3. Remove the thighs from the marinade and discard the extra marinade. Preheat the barbecue to medium. Grill the chicken for about 20 minutes, turning once, or until the internal temperature is 165°F.

Serves: 5   Prep Time: 10 mins.   Cook Time: 20 mins.

Calories: 621; Fat: 21g; Carbs: 3g; Phosphorus: 131mg; Potassium: 220mg; Sodium: 86mg; Protein: 22g

Snacks

Scrumptious Apple Bars

Stage 2: Mild damage in kidneys (eGFR = 60–89 mL)

Ingredients:

- Sugar, 1 cup, granulated
- vanilla extract, 1 tsp.
- Sugar, 1 cup, powdered
- sour cream, 1 cup
- baking soda, 1 tsp.
- brown sugar, 1/2 cup
- sea salt, 1/2 tsp.
- cinnamon, 1 tsp.
- flour, 2 cups, all-purpose
- apples, 2, medium
- milk, 2 tablespoons
- butter, 3/4 cup, unsalted

Directions:

1. Preheat the oven to 350°F. Peel and chop the apples. Cream 1/2 cup of butter and granulated sugar. Stir in flour, salt, baking soda, vanilla and sour cream. Mix well. Stir in chopped apples.

2. Pour batter into a greased 9 x 13-inch baking pan. Combine cinnamon, brown sugar and 2 tablespoons of slightly softened butter then add evenly on top of your batter. Bake for about 35 minutes then set aside to cool.

3. Create an icing by combining your milk, and melted butter then incorporate your powdered sugar until the preferred consistency is achieved. Drizzle on the top then cut slice in 18 bars.

Serves: 18   Prep Time: 15 mins.   Cook Time: 35 mins.

Calories: 481; Carbs: 29g; Protein: 2.3g; Fat: 6.72g; Phosphorus: 31mg; Potassium: 74mg; Sodium: 80mg

Day 7

Breakfast

Breakfast Banana Delight

Stage 2: Mild damage in kidneys (eGFR = 60–89 mL)

Ingredients:

- ½ tsp nutmeg
- 1 cup banana (chopped)
- 1 tbsp oil
- ¼ cup egg substitute
- ½ cup skim milk
- 1 tbsp sodium free baking powder
- 1 tbsp sugar
- 1 cup flour

Directions:

In a bowl, mix and stir baking powder, sugar and flour. In a separate bowl, combine oil, egg and milk then add nutmeg and banana. Add the mixture into the bowl of dry ingredients. In a hot frying pan, drop just by tablespoonfuls and fry for about 2 to 3 minutes. Wait until it is golden brown then drain and serve.

Serves: 4   Prep Time: 10 mins.   Cook Time: 3 mins.

Calories per Serving: 570; Carbs: 55g; Protein: 7g; Fat: 5g; Phosphorus: 350mg; Potassium: 350mg; Sodium: 48mg

Lunch

Creole Jambalaya

Stage 2: Mild damage in kidneys (eGFR = 60–89 mL)

Ingredients:

- ¼ cup Green onions
- ¼ tsp cayenne
- ¼ tsp Thyme
- ½ cup celery
- ½ cup Green bell peppers
- ½ lb. shrimp, peeled and deveined
- 1 tbsp olive oil
- 2 chicken breast halves, skinless and boneless
- 2 cups long grain rice
- 2 onions, chopped
- 2 tbsps Worcestershire
- 3 tbsps garlic, minced
- 3 whole tomatoes, chopped
- 5 cups water

Directions:

1. Bring a large saucepan, filled with 5 cups water, to a boil. Add shrimps and boil for 2 minutes. Drain shrimps, reserve liquid and transfer to a plate. In same saucepan, add the reserved liquid from shrimp, 1/3 garlic, ½ of the celery, ½ of onions, all the tomatoes and the 2 chicken breasts. Bring to a boil and once boiling, lower fire to a simmer.
2. Partially cover pan and simmer for 25 minutes or until chicken is cooked and juices run clear. Remove cooked

chicken and chop coarsely once cool to handle. As for the liquid, reserve and just add more water to reach 4 cups.

3. In a Dutch oven placed on medium high fire, heat oil. Mix in cayenne, thyme, Worcestershire sauce, tomatoes and juice, and the reserved cooking liquid. Cook for 5 minutes while stirring constantly to break up the tomatoes.

4. Add rice and bring to a simmer, once simmering lower fire to medium low, cover and cook for 25 minutes or until water is fully absorbed by the rice. Turn off fire.

5. Mix in cooked chicken and shrimps. Cover pot and allow to stand for 5 minutes more to continue cooking. To serve, transfer to serving bowls and sprinkle with parsley.

Serves:6   Prep Time: 10 mins.   Cook Time: 1 hr. 20 mins.

Calories: 519; Carbs: 57g; Protein: 35g; Fat: 14g; Phosphorus: 487mg; Potassium: 683mg; Sodium: 466mg

Dinner

Garlic Cauliflower Rice

Stage 2: Mild damage in kidneys (eGFR = 60–89 mL)

Ingredients:

- 1 medium head cauliflower
- 1 tablespoon extra-virgin olive oil
- 4 garlic cloves, minced
- Freshly ground black pepper

Directions:

1. Using a sharp knife, remove the core of the cauliflower, and separate the cauliflower into florets. In a food processor,

pulse the florets until they are the size of rice, being careful not to over process them to the point of becoming mushy.

2. Add your oil on in a skillet on medium heat. Add the garlic and stir until just fragrant. Add the cauliflower, stirring to coat. Add 1 tablespoon of water to the pan, cover, and reduce the heat to low. Steam for 7 to 10 minutes, until the cauliflower is tender. Season with pepper and serve.

Serves: 8   Prep Time: 5 mins.   Cook Time: 10 mins.

Calories: 637; Fat: 2g; Carbs: 4g; Protein: 2g; Phosphorus: 35mg; Potassium: 226mg; Sodium: 22mg

Snacks

Thai-Style Eggplant Dip

Stage 2: Mild damage in kidneys (eGFR = 60–89 mL)

Ingredients:

- 1 pound Thai eggplant (or Japanese or Chinese eggplant)
- 2 tablespoons rice vinegar
- 2 teaspoons sugar
- 1 teaspoon low-sodium soy sauce
- 1 jalapeño pepper
- 2 garlic cloves
- ¼ cup chopped basil
- Cut vegetables or crackers, for serving

Directions:

1. Preheat the oven to 425°F. Pierce the eggplant in several places with a skewer or knife. Place on a rimmed baking sheet and cook until soft, about 30 minutes. Let cool, cut in half, and scoop out the flesh of the eggplant into a blender. Add the rice vinegar, sugar, soy sauce, jalapeño, garlic, and

basil to the blender. Process until smooth. Serve with cut vegetables or crackers.

Serves: 4   Prep Time: 10 mins.   Cook Time: 30 mins.

Calories: 440; Fat: 0g; Carbs: 10g; Protein: 2g; Phosphorus: 34mg; Potassium: 284mg; Sodium: 47mg

Day 8

Breakfast

Pear, Chicken and Almond Garden Salad

Stage 2: Mild damage in kidneys (eGFR = 60–89 mL)

Ingredients:

- 2 tbsps toasted slivered almonds
- 1 head lettuce, torn to bite sized pieces, reserving 3 large leaves
- 2 fresh NW pears cut into 1-inch cubes
- ¼ tsp ground ginger
- ½ tsp prepared mustard
- 2 tbsps reduced-calorie mayonnaise
- ½ cup low fat plain yogurt
- ¼ tsp diced celery
- ½ cup green pepper, sliced lengthwise
- 2 cups cooked boneless, skinless chicken breasts sliced into ½-inch cubes

Directions:

1. In a bowl mix celery, green pepper and chicken. Season with non-iodized salt. Add ginger, mustard, mayonnaise and yogurt into bowl of chicken and mix well. Fold in pears and toss to mix.

2. Arrange 4 large lettuce leaves on 4 plates. Evenly divide and spread torn lettuce leaves inside the large lettuce leaves. Top it with ¼ of the chicken mixture, serve and enjoy.

Serves: 4   Prep Time: 10 mins.   Cook Time: 10 mins.

Calories per Serving: 542; Carbs: 17g; Protein: 8g; Fat: 6g; Phosphorus: 114 mg; Potassium: 278mg; Sodium: 190mg

Lunch

Celery and Arugula Salad

Stage 2: Mild damage in kidneys (eGFR = 60–89 mL)

Ingredients:
- 1 shallot, thinly sliced
- 3 celery stalks, cut into 1-inch pieces about ¼ inch thick
- 2 cups loosely packed arugula
- 1 tablespoon extra-virgin olive oil
- 2 tablespoons white wine vinegar
- Freshly ground black pepper
- 2 tablespoons grated Parmesan cheese

Directions:
1. In a medium bowl, toss the shallot, celery stalks, and arugula. In a small bowl, whisk the olive oil, vinegar, and pepper.
2. Toss your salad with your dressing. Top with Parmesan cheese and serve.

Serves: 4   Prep Time: 10 mins.   Cook Time: 0 mins.

Calories: 545; Fat: 4g; Carbs: 1g; Protein: 1g; Phosphorus: 23mg; Potassium: 47mg; Sodium: 47mg

Dinner

Chicken Breast and Bok Choy in Parchment

Stage 2: Mild damage in kidneys (eGFR = 60–89 mL)

Ingredients:

- 1 tablespoon Dijon mustard
- 1 tablespoon extra-virgin olive oil
- 1 tablespoon chopped fresh thyme leaves
- 2 cups thinly sliced bok choy
- 2 carrots, julienned
- 1 small leek, thinly sliced
- 4 boneless, skinless chicken breasts
- Freshly ground black pepper
- 4 lemon slices

Directions:

1. Preheat the oven to 425°F. In a small bowl, mix the mustard, olive oil, and thyme. Prepare four pieces of parchment paper by folding four 18-inch pieces in half and cutting them like you would to create a heart. Open each piece and lay flat.
2. In each piece of parchment, arrange ½ cup of bok choy, a small handful of carrots, and a few slices of leek. Place the chicken breast on top, and season with pepper. Brush the marinade over the chicken breasts, and top each with a slice of lemon.
3. Fold the packets shut, and fold the paper along the edges to crease and seal the packages. Cook for 20 minutes. Let rest for 5 minutes, and open carefully to serve.

Serves: 4   Prep Time: 10 mins.   Cook Time: 30 mins.

Calories: 564; Fat: 5g; Carbs: 8g; Protein: 24g; Phosphorus: 26mg; Potassium: 187mg; Sodium: 356mg

Snacks

Pineapple Raspberry Parfaits

Stage 2: Mild damage in kidneys (eGFR = 60–89 mL)

Ingredients:

½ pint fresh raspberries
1 ½ cup fresh or frozen pineapple chunks
2 8oz containers non-fat peach yogurt

Directions:

1. In a parfait glass, layer the yogurt, raspberries and pineapples alternately. Chill inside the refrigerator. Serve chilled.

Serves: 2   Prep Time: 6 mins.   Cook Time: 0 mins.

Calories: 619; Carbs: 60g; Protein: 22g; Fat: 1g; Phosphorus: 293mg; Potassium: 479mg; Sodium: 85mg

Day 9

Breakfast

Egg And Veggie Muffins

Stage 2: Mild damage in kidneys (eGFR = 60–89 mL)

Ingredients:

51

- Cooking spray, for greasing the muffin pans
- 4 eggs
- 2 tablespoons unsweetened rice milk
- ½ sweet onion, finely chopped
- ½ red bell pepper, finely chopped
- 1 tablespoon chopped fresh parsley
- Pinch red pepper flakes
- Pinch freshly ground black pepper

Directions:

1. Preheat the oven to 350°F.Spray 4 muffin pans with cooking spray; set aside. In a large bowl, whisk together the eggs, milk, onion, red pepper, parsley, red pepper flakes, and black pepper until well combined.
2. Pour the egg mixture into the prepared muffin pans. Bake 18 to 20 minutes or until the muffins are puffed and golden. Serve warm or cold.

Serves: 4   Prep Time: 15 mins.   Cook Time: 20 mins.

Calories: 484; Fat: 5g; Carbs: 3g; Phosphorus: 110mg; Potassium: 117mg; Sodium: 75mg; Protein: 7g

Lunch

Roasted Beet Salad

Stage 2: Mild damage in kidneys (eGFR = 60–89 mL)
Ingredients:

- 8 small beets, trimmed
- 2 tablespoons plus 1 teaspoon extra-virgin olive oil, divided
- 1 tablespoon white wine vinegar
- 1 teaspoon Dijon mustard
- Freshly ground black pepper

- 4 cups baby salad greens
- ½ sweet onion, sliced
- 2 tablespoons crumbled feta cheese
- 2 tablespoons walnut pieces

Directions:

1. Preheat the oven to 400°F.Toss the beets with 1 teaspoon of olive oil, wrap them in aluminum foil, and cook for 30 minutes, until fork-tender. Put 2 tablespoons of olive oil, mustard and apple cider vinegar in a bowl. Season with pepper.
2. In a medium bowl, mix the salad greens, onion, feta cheese, and walnuts. Toss with about half of the vinaigrette. Arrange on four plates. Slice the beets into wedges and top the salads. Serve with the remaining dressing.
3.

Serves: 4   Prep Time: 10 mins.   Cook Time: 30 mins.

Calories: 570; Fat: 9g; Carbs: 20g; Protein: 4g; Phosphorus: 93mg; Potassium: 585mg; Sodium: 217mg

Dinner

Indian Chicken Curry

Stage 2: Mild damage in kidneys (eGFR = 60–89 mL)

Ingredients:

- 3 tablespoons olive oil, divided
- 6 boneless, skinless chicken thighs
- 1 small sweet onion
- 2 teaspoons minced garlic
- 1 teaspoon grated fresh ginger
- 1 tablespoon Hot Curry Powder (here)
- ¾ cup water
- ¼ cup coconut milk
- 2 tablespoons chopped fresh cilantro

Directions:

1. In a large skillet over a medium-high heat, heat 2 tablespoons of the oil. Add the chicken and cook for about 10 minutes or until the thighs are browned all over. With tongs, remove the chicken to a plate and set aside.
2. Add the remaining 1 tablespoon of oil to the skillet and sauté the onion, garlic, and ginger for about 3 minutes or until they are softened. Stir in the curry powder, water, and coconut milk.
3. Return the chicken to the skillet and bring the liquid to a boil. Reduce the heat to low, cover the skillet, and simmer for about 25 minutes or until the chicken is tender and the sauce is thick. Serve topped with cilantro.

Serves: 6   Prep Time: 20 mins.   Cook Time: 40 mins.

Calories: 441; Fat: 14g; Carbs: 2g; Phosphorus: 145mg; Potassium: 230mg; Sodium: 76mg; Protein: 26g

Snacks

Simple Roasted Broccoli

Stage 2: Mild damage in kidneys (eGFR = 60–89 mL)

Ingredients:

- 2 small heads broccoli, cut into florets
- 1 tablespoon extra-virgin olive oil
- 3 garlic cloves, minced

Directions:

1. Preheat the oven to 425°F. In a medium bowl, toss the broccoli with the olive oil and garlic. Spread evenly on a baking tray in a single layer. Roast for 10 minutes, then flip the broccoli and roast an additional 10 minutes. Serve.

Serves: 6   Prep Time: 5 mins.   Cook Time: 20 mins.

Calories: 538; Fat: 2g; Carbs: 4g; Protein: 1g; Phosphorus: 32mg; Potassium: 150mg; Sodium: 15mg

Day 10

Breakfast

Poppy Seed-Lemon Dressing on Winter Fruit Salad

Stage 2: Mild damage in kidneys (eGFR = 60–89 mL)

Ingredients:

- 1 pear, peeled, cored and diced
- 1 apple, peeled cored and diced
- ¼ cup dried cranberries
- 1 cup cashews
- 4 oz shredded Swiss cheese
- Romaine lettuce, 1 head, torn
- 1 tbsp poppy seeds
- 2/3 cup vegetable oil
- ½ tsp sea salt
- 1 tsp Dijon-style prepared mustard
- 2 tsps diced onion
- ½ cup lemon juice
- ½ cup white sugar

Directions:

1. In blender, process salt, mustard, onion, lemon juice, and sugar until smooth and creamy. Slowly pour in oil as blender is running. Continue blending until smooth and creamy. Add poppy seeds, blend one more time and set aside.

2. Mix well cubed pear, cubes apple, cranberries, cashews, Swiss cheese and lettuce in a large salad bowl. Pour in dressing, toss well to coat.

   Serves: 8   Prep Time: 15 mins.   Cook Time: 0 mins.

Calories: 534; Carbs: 20g; Protein: 7g; Fat: 28g; Phosphorus: 172mg; Potassium: 409mg; Sodium: 177mg

Lunch

Summer Pasta Salad with White Wine Vinaigrette

Stage 2: Mild damage in kidneys (eGFR = 60–89 mL)

Ingredients:

- 1 pound small pasta noodles (such as penne, farfalle, elbow, or rotini)
- 1 large cucumber, cut lengthwise and sliced into half moons
- 2 cups arugula, coarsely chopped
- 3 garlic cloves, minced
- 2 tablespoons extra-virgin olive oil
- 1 tablespoon white wine vinegar
- Freshly ground black pepper
- ¼ cup grated Parmesan cheese

Directions:

1. Fill a large stockpot halfway with water and bring to a boil. Add the pasta and cook until al dente. Drain then use cold water on the pasta to stop the cooking. In a large bowl, toss the noodles, cucumber, arugula, and garlic. Drizzle the olive oil and vinegar over the salad, and season with pepper. Stir in the Parmesan cheese and serve.

   Serves: 8   Prep Time: 10 mins.   Cook Time: 15 mins.

Calories: 527; Fat: 4g; Carbs: 43g; Protein: 9g; Phosphorus: 36mg; Potassium: 82mg; Sodium: 60mg

Dinner

Thai-Style Chicken Curry

Stage 2: Mild damage in kidneys (eGFR = 60–89 mL)

Ingredients:

For the curry paste:

- 2 dried Thai red chiles
- 2 teaspoons coriander seeds
- 1 lemongrass stalk, outer layer removed, ends trimmed, tender green and white parts minced
- 1 shallot
- 4 garlic cloves
- 2-inch piece ginger, thinly sliced
- ½ cup coarsely chopped fresh cilantro leaves and stems
- 1 teaspoon low-sodium soy sauce
- 2 tablespoons lime juice

For the curry:

- 1 teaspoon canola oil
- 1 pound boneless, skinless chicken breast, thinly sliced
- 1 cup green beans, cut into 2-inch segments
- 1 cup water
- Juice of 1 lime
- 1 teaspoon brown sugar

Directions:

To make the curry paste:

1. In a small bowl, add the chiles and cover with hot water. Leave to soak for 10 minutes. Meanwhile, in a small, dry

57

skillet, toast the coriander seeds until fragrant, shaking the pan constantly to prevent burning. Transfer immediately to a food processor.

2. Drain the chiles and add them to the food processor, then add the lemongrass, shallot, garlic, ginger, cilantro, soy sauce, and lime juice. Grind into a fine paste, adding 1 or 2 tablespoons of water if needed. Use immediately, or transfer to an airtight container and store refrigerated for up to three days.

To make the curry:

1. In a large skillet or wok over medium-high heat, heat the oil. Add the curry paste, and cook, stirring constantly, for about 30 seconds, until fragrant. Add the chicken breast, and stir continuously until just browned.

2. Add the beans and 1 cup of water. Simmer for 5 minutes, until the chicken is cooked through and the vegetables are tender. Season with the lime juice and brown sugar. Serve over rice or rice noodles.

Serves: 4   Prep Time: 15 mins.   Cook Time: 15 mins.

Calories: 449; Fat: 3g; Carbs: 9g; Protein: 25g; Phosphorus: 35mg; Potassium: 205mg; Sodium: 280mg

Snacks

Roasted Red Pepper Hummus

Stage 2: Mild damage in kidneys (eGFR = 60–89 mL)

Ingredients:

- 1 red bell pepper
- 1 (15-ounce) can chickpeas, drained and rinsed
- Juice of 1 lemon
- 2 tablespoons tahini
- 2 garlic cloves

- 2 tablespoons extra-virgin olive oil

Directions:

1. Move an oven rack to the highest position. Heat the broiler to high. Core the pepper and cut it into three or four large pieces. Arrange them on a baking sheet, skin-side up.
2. Broil the peppers for 5 to 10 minutes, until the skins are charred. Remove from the oven and transfer the peppers to a small bowl. Cover with plastic wrap and let them steam for 10 to 15 minutes, until cool enough to handle.
3. Peel the charred skin off the peppers, and place the peppers in a blender. Add the chickpeas, lemon juice, tahini, garlic, and olive oil. Process until smooth, adding up to 1 tablespoon of water to adjust consistency as desired.

Serves: 8   Prep Time: 10 mins.   Cook Time: 10 mins.

Calories: 503; Fat: 6g; Carbs: 10g; Protein: 3g; Phosphorus: 58mg; Potassium: 91mg; Sodium: 72mg

Day 11

Breakfast

Baked Oatmeal with Apple Spice Flavor

Stage 2: Mild damage in kidneys (eGFR = 60–89 mL)

Ingredients:

- 2 tbsps chopped nuts
- 2 tbsps brown sugar
- 1 tsp cinnamon
- ¼ tsp sea salt
- 2 cups rolled oats
- 1 apple, chopped
- 2 tbsps oil

- 1 tsp vanilla
- 1 ½ cups non-fat milk
- ½ cup applesauce, sweetened
- 1 egg, beaten

Directions:

1. With cooking spray, grease an 8 x 8-inch baking pan and preheat oven to 375oF. In a large bowl, mix oil, vanilla, milk, applesauce and egg. Thoroughly mix. In a medium bowl, combine cinnamon, salt, baking powder and rolled oats.
2. Pour the dry ingredients into the bowl of wet ingredients and mix well. Transfer batter into prepped pan and spread evenly. Set to bake until done. (about 25 minutes).
3. Remove from oven and sprinkle with nuts and brown sugar. Return to oven and broil for 3 to 4 minutes or until top of oats be bubbly. Remove from oven; let it cool before slicing into 9 equal squares. You can serve right away or store in tightly lidded containers for up to 5 days.

Serves: 6   Prep Time: 15 mins.   Cook Time: 40 mins.

Calories: 573; Carbs: 36g; Protein: 9g; Fat: 6g; Phosphorus: 312mg; Potassium: 333mg; Sodium: 146mg

Lunch

Easy Baked Shepherd's Pie

Stage 2: Mild damage in kidneys (eGFR = 60–89 mL)

Ingredients:

- Pepper to taste
- ½ cup shredded cheddar cheese
- ¾ cup reduced sodium chicken broth
- 4 cups frozen mixed vegetables
- 2 tbsps flour
- 1 clove garlic, minced
- 1 medium onion, chopped
- 1 lb. lean ground chicken

- ½ cup low fat milk
- 2 large baking potatoes, peeled and diced

Directions:

1. In a saucepan, bring to boil potatoes with water barely covering it. Once boiling, reduce fire to a simmer and cook for 15 minutes or until soft while covered. Once soft, drain potatoes, transfer to a bowl and mash. Add milk and mix well.
2. Preheat oven to 375oF. In a large skillet, grease with cooking spray and sauté garlic and onions for a minute. Add ground chicken and sauté until brown around 8 to 10 minutes. Add flour and sauté for another minute.
3. Add broth and mixed vegetables. Sauté until bubbly, around 5 minutes. Transfer mixture into an 8-inch square baking dish. Cover the top with mashed potato mixture and sprinkle cheese on top. Pop into the oven and bake until bubbly around 25 minutes. Serve and enjoy.

Serves: 6   Prep Time: 10 mins.   Cook Time: 25 mins.

Calories: 1639; Carbs: 27g; Protein: 31g; Fat: 163g; Phosphorus: 425mg; Potassium: 896mg; Sodium: 419mg

Dinner

Chickpeas Soup Moroccan Style

Stage 2: Mild damage in kidneys (eGFR = 60–89 mL)

Ingredients:

- 2 handfuls baby spinach
- 1 tbsp tomato paste, no added salt
- ¼ tsp ground coriander
- ¼ tsp cumin
- ¼ tsp paprika, smoked or sweet
- 1 carrot, diced
- ¼ tsp chili

61

- 1 can chickpeas, drained and rinsed
- 1 clove garlic
- ½ lemon juiced and zested
- 1 large tomato, diced
- 1 cup water
- 2 cups stock
- 2 celery sticks, sliced
- 1 onion, diced
- 1 tbsp olive oil

Directions:

1. On medium high fire, place a soup pot and heat oil. Add onions and sauté for 3 minutes. Add carrot, chili and celery. For 3 minutes more, continue sautéing. Add garlic, paprika, coriander, and cumin. Cook for a minute. Add chickpeas, lemon juice and zest, tomato, water and stock.
2. Bring to a boil and once simmering slow fire to low. While covered, simmer soup for 20 minutes. Add tomato paste and baby spinach. Continue simmering for another ten minutes. Ladle soup to serving bowls and best enjoyed with a side of crusty bread.

Serves: 4   Prep Time: 20 mins.   Cook Time: 40 mins.

Calories: 569; Carbs: 22g; Protein: 10g; Fat: 6g; Phosphorus: 209mg; Potassium: 1039mg; Sodium: 282mg

Snacks

Almond Walnut Granola

Stage 2: Mild damage in kidneys (eGFR = 60–89 mL)

Ingredients:

- ¼ cup canola oil
- ½ cup unsweetened coconut, shredded
- ¾ cups walnuts, chopped
- 1 ½ tsp vanilla

- 1 cup almonds, slivered
- 1 cup raisins
- 2 cups bran flakes
- 4 tbsp honey
- 6 cups rolled oats (old fashioned)

Directions:

1. Prepare a baking sheet by lightly spraying with cooking spray and preheat oven to 325oF. On low fire, place a small saucepan and add vanilla, honey and oil. Cook for 5 minutes while stirring occasionally to combine thoroughly.
2. In a large mixing bowl, thoroughly combine walnuts, bran flakes, coconut, almonds, and oats. Pour in the honey mixture while mixing to coat ingredients evenly.
3. Spread mixture in an even layer on baking tray, pop in the oven and bake until lightly browned and crisped. This will take around 25 minutes of baking. Remove from oven and cool. Once cooled, mix in raisins. One serving is equal to a half cup.

Serves: 24   Prep Time: 15 mins.   Cook Time: 30 mins.

Calories: 354; Carbs: 23g; Protein: 6g; Fat: 9g; Phosphorus: 228mg; Potassium: 206mg; Sodium: 33mg

Day 12

Breakfast

Sandwich with Spinach and Tuna Salad

Stage 3: Moderate damage in kidneys (eGFR = 30–59 mL)

Stage 4: Severe damage in kidneys (eGFR = 15–29 mL)

Ingredients:

- 1 cup fresh baby spinach
- 8 slices 100% whole wheat sandwich bread
- ¼ tsp freshly ground black pepper
- ½ tsp salt free seasoning blend
- Juice of one lemon
- 2 tbsps olive oil
- ½ tsp dill weed
- 2 ribs celery, diced

Directions:
1. In a medium bowl, mix well dill weed, celery, onion, cucumber and tuna. Add lemon juice and olive oil and mix thoroughly. Season with pepper and salt-free seasoning blend.
2. To assemble sandwich, you can toast bread slices, on top of one bread slice layer ½ cup tuna salad, top with ¼ cup spinach and cover with another slice of bread. Repeat procedure to remaining ingredients, serve and enjoy.

Serves: 4   Prep Time: 15 mins.   Cook Time: 0 mins.

Calories: 320; Carbs: 49g; Protein: 9g; Fat: 12g; Phosphorus: 177mg; Potassium: 347mg; Sodium: 615mg

Lunch

Quick Thai Chicken and Vegetable Curry

Stage 3: Moderate damage in kidneys (eGFR = 30–59 mL)

Stage 4: Severe damage in kidneys (eGFR = 15–29 mL)

Ingredients:
- 1 ½ cups cauliflower florets
- 1 clove garlic, minced
- 1 cup light coconut milk

- 1 cup low sodium chicken broth
- 1 lb chicken breasts
- 1 medium bell pepper, julienned
- 1 medium onion, halved and sliced
- 1 tbsp fish sauce or low sodium soy sauce
- 1 tbsp fresh ginger, minced
- 1 tbsp lime juice
- 1 tsp light brown sugar
- 1 tsp red curry paste
- 2 cups baby spinach
- 2 tsp canola oil
- Lime wedges

Directions:

1. Heat oil in a skillet over medium high flame. Sauté the onion and bell pepper for four minutes or until soft. Add the ginger, garlic and curry paste. Mix then add the chicken. Sauté for two minutes before adding the coconut milk, broth, brown sugar and fish sauce.
2. Add the cauliflowers and reduce the heat to medium low. Simmer and stir the mixture occasionally until the chicken is cooked through. Add the spinach and lime juice and cook until the spinach has wilted. Serve immediately with lime wedges.

Serves: 4   Prep Time: 15 mins.   Cook Time: 20 mins.
Calories: 594; Carbs: 11g; Protein: 29g; Fat: 28g; Phosphorus: 316mg; Potassium: 745mg; Sodium: 252mg

Dinner

Chicken Satay with Peanut Sauce

Stage 3: Moderate damage in kidneys (eGFR = 30–59 mL)

Stage 4: Severe damage in kidneys (eGFR = 15–29 mL)

Ingredients:

For the chicken:

- ½ cup plain, unsweetened yogurt
- 2 garlic cloves, minced
- 1-inch piece ginger, minced
- 2 teaspoons curry powder
- 1 lb. chicken breast, skinless, boneless, cut into strips
- 1 teaspoon canola oil

For the peanut sauce:

- ¾ cup smooth unsalted peanut butter
- 1 teaspoon soy sauce
- 1 tablespoon brown sugar
- Juice of 2 limes
- ½ teaspoon red chili flakes
- ¼ cup hot water
- Fresh cilantro leaves, chopped, for garnish
- Lime wedges, for garnish

Directions:

To make the chicken:

1. In a small bowl, add the yogurt, garlic, ginger, and curry powder. Stir to mix. Add the chicken strips to the marinade. Cover and refrigerate for 2 hours. Thread the chicken pieces onto skewers. Brush a grill pan with the oil, and heat on medium-high. Cook the chicken skewers on each side for 3 to 5 minutes, until cooked through.

   To make the peanut sauce:

2. In a food processor, combine the peanut butter, soy sauce, brown sugar, lime juice, red chili flakes, and hot water. Process until smooth. Transfer to a bowl, and sprinkle with the cilantro. Serve with the chicken satay along with lime wedges for squeezing over the skewers.

Serves: 6   Prep Time: 10 mins.   Cook Time: 10 mins.

Calories: 586; Fat: 18g; Carbs: 10g; Protein: 25g; Phosphorus: 33mg; Potassium: 66mg; Sodium: 201mg

Snacks
Vegetable Couscous

Stage 3: Moderate damage in kidneys (eGFR = 30–59 mL)

Stage 4: Severe damage in kidneys (eGFR = 15–29 mL)

Ingredients:

- 1 tablespoon extra-virgin olive oil
- ½ sweet onion, diced
- 1 carrot, diced
- 1 celery stalk, diced
- ½ cup diced red or yellow bell pepper
- 1 small zucchini, diced
- 1 cup couscous
- 1½ cups Simple Chicken Broth or low-sodium store-bought chicken stock
- ½ teaspoon garlic powder
- Freshly ground black pepper

Directions:

1. Set your oil on in a skillet on medium heat. Add the onion, carrot, celery, and bell pepper, and cook, stirring occasionally, until the vegetables are just becoming tender, about 5 to 7 minutes.

2. Add the zucchini, couscous, broth, and garlic powder. Stir to blend, and bring to a boil. Cover and remove from the heat. Let stand for 5 to 8 minutes. Fluff with a fork, season with pepper, and serve.

Serves: 6   Prep Time: 10 mins.   Cook Time: 15 mins.

Calories: 454; Fat: 3g; Carbs: 27g; Protein: 5g; Phosphorus: 83mg; Potassium: 197mg; Sodium: 36mg

Day 13

Breakfast

Quinoa, Cilantro and Cranberry Salad

Stage 3: Moderate damage in kidneys (eGFR = 30–59 mL)
Stage 4: Severe damage in kidneys (eGFR = 15–29 mL)

Ingredients:

- ¼ cup toasted sliced almonds
- Pepper to taste
- ¼ cup yellow bell pepper, chopped
- 1 ½ cups water
- 1 cup uncooked quinoa, rinsed
- 1 small red onion, finely chopped
- 1 ½ tsp curry powder
- ½ cup minced carrots
- ¼ cup chopped fresh cilantro
- 1 lime, juiced
- ½ cup dried cranberries
- ¼ cup red bell pepper, chopped
- 1/8 tsp sea salt

Directions:

1. Boil the water in the pan and add quinoa. Let it cook for 20 minutes. The salad bowl should hold the quinoa and then put it into the refrigerator.
2. After 45 - 60 minutes add the almonds, cranberries, curry, onion, lime juice and pepper into the bowl. Put the bowl

back to the refrigerator for another 45 - 60 minutes before serving.

Serves: 6   Prep Time: 15 mins.   Cook Time: 1 hr. 20 mins.

Calories: 449; Carbs: 25g; Protein: 5g; Fat: 3g; Phosphorus: 145mg; Potassium: 263mg; Sodium: 63mg

Lunch

Mexican Baked Beans and Rice

Stage 3: Moderate damage in kidneys (eGFR = 30–59 mL)
Stage 4: Severe damage in kidneys (eGFR = 15–29 mL)
Ingredients:

- 1 cup shredded reduced fat Monterey Jack cheese
- 4 garlic cloves, crushed
- 1 tbsp cumin
- 1 tbsp chili powder
- 1 cup chopped poblano pepper
- 1 cup chopped red bell pepper
- 1 cup frozen yellow corn
- black beans, (15-oz, no-salt added) drained and rinsed
- 2 14.5-oz cans no salt added tomatoes, diced or crushed
- 1 lb. chicken breast, skinless, boneless, cubed
- 1 ½ cups cooked brown rice

Directions:

1. With cooking spray grease a 3-quart shallow casserole and preheat oven to 400oF. Spread cooked brown rice in bottom of casserole. Layer chicken on top of brown rice.
2. Mix well garlic, seasonings, peppers, corn, beans and tomatoes in a medium bowl. Evenly spread bean mixture on top of chicken. Sprinkle cheese on top of beans and pop into the oven. Set to bake until cooked (about 45 minutes). Switch off oven and serve.

   Serves: 6   Prep Time: 20 mins.   Cook Time: 1 hr.

Calories: 564; Carbs: 22g; Protein: 27g; Fat: 9g; Phosphorus: 353mg; Potassium: 682mg; Sodium: 280mg

Dinner

Turkey Meatballs and Spaghetti in Garlic Sauce

Stage 3: Moderate damage in kidneys (eGFR = 30–59 mL)
Stage 4: Severe damage in kidneys (eGFR = 15–29 mL)

Ingredients:

For the meatballs:
- ¾ pound lean ground turkey
- ½ cup bread crumbs
- 1 large egg, beaten
- ½ teaspoon onion powder
- ½ teaspoon garlic powder

For the pasta:
- 8 ounces spaghetti noodles
- 1 tablespoon extra-virgin olive oil
- 5 garlic cloves, minced
- 2 cups chopped broccoli rabe
- ¼ cup shredded Parmesan cheese
- Freshly ground black pepper

-

Directions:

To make the meatballs:
1. Heat the oven to 375°F. Line a baking sheet with parchment paper. In a medium bowl, combine the turkey, breadcrumbs, egg, onion powder, and garlic powder. Mix well.
2. Shape the turkey mixture into 2-inch round meatballs and place them on the baking sheet. Bake for 20 minutes, until

70

browned and cooked through, flipping the meatballs once halfway through cooking.

To make the pasta:

1. Bring a pot of water to a boil and cook the noodles al dente. Set aside a cup of your cooking liquid then discard the remainder. Set your oil to heat in a skillet on medium heat.
2. Add the garlic and cook until fragrant. Add ½ cup of the reserved cooking water and broccoli rabe to the skillet. To simmer ensure that the heat is reduced, and cook for 5 minutes while covered, until the broccoli rabe is fork-tender.
3. Add the noodles to the skillet and mix. Add a couple of tablespoons or more of the remaining cooking water to the skillet, to wet the noodles. Stir in the Parmesan cheese and season with pepper. Serve the noodles topped with the meatballs.

Serves: 4   Prep Time: 15 mins.   Cook Time: 20 mins.

Calories: 450; Fat: 15g; Carbs: 55g; Protein: 23g; Phosphorus: 319mg; Potassium: 354mg; Sodium: 245mg

Snacks

Pumpkin Walnut Cookie

Stage 3: Moderate damage in kidneys (eGFR = 30–59 mL)
Stage 4: Severe damage in kidneys (eGFR = 15–29 mL)

Ingredients:

- ½ cup olive oil
- 1 ½ cups brown sugar
- 1 ¾ cups pumpkin, cooked and pureed (15 oz. can)
- 1 cup raisin
- 1 cup walnuts or hazelnuts, chopped
- 1 tbsp baking powder
- 1¼ cups whole wheat flour

71

- 1½ cups flour
- 1½ tsp pumpkin pie spice mix
- 2 eggs

Directions:

1. Grease a cookie sheet with cooking spray and preheat oven to 400°F. In a medium bowl mix baking powder, sea salt, pumpkin pie spice mix, whole wheat flour and flour. In a large bowl beat eggs and oil thoroughly.
2. Add in brown sugar and beat for at least 3 minutes. Mix in pumpkin puree and beat well. Slowly add the dry ingredients beating well after each addition.
3. Fold in nuts and raisins. Using a 1 tbsp measuring spoon, get a tablespoon full of the dough and place on cookie sheet at least 2-inches apart.
4. With the bottom of a spoon, flatten cookie. Pop into the oven and bake until golden brown, around 10-12 minutes. Once done, remove from oven, serve and enjoy or store in tightly lidded containers for up to a week.

Serves: 48   Prep Time: 10 mins.   Cook Time: 15 mins.

Calories: 513; Carbs: 15g; Protein: 3g; Fat: 5g; Phosphorus: 71mg; Potassium: 125mg; Sodium: 17mg

Day 14

Breakfast

Pasta with Parmesan Broccoli Sauce

Stage 3: Moderate damage in kidneys (eGFR = 30–59 mL)

Stage 4: Severe damage in kidneys (eGFR = 15–29 mL)

Ingredients:

- Pepper and sea salt to taste
- 2 tbsps olive oil, divided
- ¼ cup grated Parmesan cheese

- 5 cloves garlic, smashed and chopped
- 6 ½ cups fresh broccoli florets, no stems
- 12-oz uncooked whole wheat pasta

Directions:

1. In a large pot of boiling water, cook pasta according to manufacturer's instructions. 5 minutes before pasta is done, add broccoli into pot, cover and cook until pasta is done.
2. Drain pasta and broccoli, while reserving 1 cup of liquid. Separate broccoli from pasta. Return pot into high fire and heat oil. Sauté garlic until lightly browned.
3. Lower fire to medium and return broccoli. Season with pepper and salt to taste. Add cheese and water, mix until well combined. Turn off fire and transfer broccoli mixture into blender. Puree until smooth and creamy.
4. Return to pot and turn on fire to medium and add pasta back. Cook until well combined and heated through around 5 to 10 minutes. Serve and enjoy.

Serves: 6   Prep Time: 10 mins.   Cook Time: 1 hr.

Calories: 522; Carbs: 46g; Protein: 9g; Fat: 3g; Phosphorus: 248mg; Potassium: 351mg; Sodium: 22mg

Lunch

Pear and Watercress Salad

Stage 3: Moderate damage in kidneys (eGFR = 30–59 mL)

Stage 4: Severe damage in kidneys (eGFR = 15–29 mL)

Ingredients:
- ¼ cup sweet onion, coarsely chopped
- 1 teaspoon Dijon mustard
- 2 tablespoons extra-virgin olive oil

- 1 tablespoon white wine vinegar
- 1 teaspoon honey
- 1 bunch watercress, thick stems removed, washed well
- 2 ripe pears, cored and cut into wedges
- 1 ounce crumbled feta cheese

Directions:

1. In a food processor or blender, combine the onion, mustard, olive oil, vinegar, and honey. Process until smooth. In a medium bowl, toss the watercress with the dressing. Arrange on four plates. Top each with pear slices and crumbled feta cheese.

Serves: 4   Prep Time: 10 mins.   Cook Time: 0 mins.

Calories: 644; Fat: 8g Carbs: 17g; Protein: 3g; Phosphorus: 70mg; Potassium: 310mg; Sodium: 134mg

Dinner

Chicken Stir-Fry

Stage 3: Moderate damage in kidneys (eGFR = 30–59 mL)

Stage 4: Severe damage in kidneys (eGFR = 15–29 mL)

Ingredients:

- 3 tablespoons pineapple juice
- 1 tablespoon balsamic vinegar
- 1 teaspoon grated fresh ginger
- 1 teaspoon minced garlic
- 2 teaspoons cornstarch
- 2 tablespoons olive oil

- 12 ounces boneless, skinless chicken breast, cut into 1-inch chunks
- ½ cup cauliflower florets
- ½ cup carrots, cut into thin disks
- ½ cup green beans
- 3 cups cooked white rice

Directions:

1. In a small bowl, stir together the pineapple juice, balsamic vinegar, garlic, ginger, and cornstarch; set aside. In a large skillet or wok over medium-high heat, heat the olive oil. Sauté the chicken for about 6 minutes or until it is just cooked through.
2. Remove the cooked chicken to a plate. Add the cauliflower, carrots, and green beans to the skillet and stir-fry for about 4 minutes or until the vegetables are crisp and tender.
3. Return the chicken to the skillet and toss to combine. Push the chicken and vegetables over to the side of the skillet and pour the sauce into the empty spot. Cook for about 2 minutes, stirring, or until the sauce is thickened. Stir the vegetables and chicken back into the sauce to coat. Serve over rice.

Serves: 5   Prep Time: 20 mins.   Cook Time: 15 mins.
Calories: 561; Fat: 5g; Carbs: 18g; Phosphorus: 96mg; Potassium: 208mg; Sodium: 90mg; Protein: 11g

Snacks
Collard Salad Rolls with Peanut Dipping Sauce

Stage 3: Moderate damage in kidneys (eGFR = 30–59 mL)

Stage 4: Severe damage in kidneys (eGFR = 15–29 mL)

Ingredients:

For the dipping sauce:
- ¼ cup peanut butter
- 2 tablespoons honey
- Juice of 1 lime
- ¼ teaspoon red chili flakes

For the salad rolls:
- 4 ounces extra-firm tofu
- 1 bunch collard greens
- 1 cup thinly sliced purple cabbage
- 1 cup bean sprouts
- 2 carrots, cut into matchsticks
- ½ cup cilantro leaves and stems

Directions:

To make the dipping sauce:

1. In a blender, combine the peanut butter, honey, lime juice, and chili flakes, and process until smooth. Add 1 to 2 tablespoons of water as desired for consistency.

To make the salad rolls:

2. Using paper towels, press the excess moisture from the tofu. Cut into ½-inch-thick matchsticks. Remove any tough stems from the collard greens and set aside. Arrange all of the ingredients within reach. Cup one collard green leaf in your hand, and add a couple pieces of the tofu and a small amount each of the cabbage, bean sprouts, and carrots.

3. Top with a couple cilantro sprigs, and roll into a cylinder. Place each roll, seam-side down, on a serving platter while you assemble the rest of the rolls. Serve with the dipping sauce.

Serves: 4   Prep Time: 15 mins.   Cook Time: 20 mins.

Calories: 574; Fat: 9g; Carbs: 20g; Protein: 8g; Phosphorus: 56mg; Potassium: 284mg; Sodium: 42mg

Day 15

Breakfast

Slow Cooked Breakfast Oatmeal

Stage 3: Moderate damage in kidneys (eGFR = 30–59 mL)

Stage 4: Severe damage in kidneys (eGFR = 15–29 mL)

Ingredients:

- 1 tsp cinnamon
- 1 tsp molasses
- 1/3 cup dried apricots, chopped
- 1/3 cup dried cherries
- 1/3 cup raisins
- 2 cups steel-cut oats
- 4 cups water
- 4 cups fat-free milk

Directions:

1. Place all ingredients in a slow cooker. On low settings, cook oatmeal while covered for 8 to 9 hours. When done, equally transfer into bowls, serve and enjoy.

Serves: 8   Prep Time: 10 mins.   Cook Time: 8 hrs.

Calories per Serving: 421; Carbs: 27g; Protein: 9g; Fat: 2g; Phosphorus: 303mg; Potassium: 425mg; Sodium: 69mg

Lunch

Chicken, Charred Tomato and Broccoli Salad

Stage 3: Moderate damage in kidneys (eGFR = 30–59 mL)

Stage 4: Severe damage in kidneys (eGFR = 15–29 mL)

Ingredients:

- ¼ cup lemon juice
- ½ tsp chili powder
- 1 ½ lbs. boneless chicken breast
- 1 ½ lbs. medium tomato
- 1 tsp freshly ground pepper
- 1 tsp sea salt
- 4 cups broccoli florets
- 5 tbsp extra virgin olive oil, divided to 2 and 3 tablespoons

Directions:

1. Place the chicken in a skillet and add just enough water to cover the chicken. Bring to a simmer over high heat. Reduce the heat once the liquid boils and cook the chicken thoroughly for 12 minutes. Once cooked, shred the chicken into bite-sized pieces.
2. On a large pot, bring water to a boil and add the broccoli. Cook for 5 minutes until slightly tender. Drain and rinse the broccoli with cold water. Set aside. Core the tomatoes and cut them crosswise. Discard the seeds and set the tomatoes cut-side down on paper towels. Pat them dry.
3. In a heavy skillet, heat the pan over high heat until very hot. Brush the cut sides of the tomatoes with olive oil and place

them on the pan. Cook the tomatoes until the sides are charred. Set aside.

4. In the same pan, heat the remaining 3 tablespoon olive oil over medium heat. Stir the salt, chili powder and pepper and stir for 45 seconds. Pour over the lemon juice and remove the pan from the heat. Plate the broccoli, shredded chicken and chili powder mixture dressing.

Serves: 6   Prep Time: 10 mins.   Cook Time: 30 mins.

Calories: 577; Carbs: 6g; Protein: 28g; Fat: 9g; Phosphorus: 292mg; Potassium: 719mg; Sodium: 560mg

Dinner

Baked Herbed Chicken

Stage 3: Moderate damage in kidneys (eGFR = 30–59 mL)

Stage 4: Severe damage in kidneys (eGFR = 15–29 mL)

Ingredients:

- 4 garlic cloves, minced
- 1 tablespoon chopped fresh oregano
- 1 tablespoon chopped fresh parsley
- 1 teaspoon lemon zest
- 6 bone-in chicken thighs
- ¼ teaspoon freshly ground black pepper

Directions:

1. Preheat the oven to 425°F. In a small bowl, add the butter, garlic, oregano, parsley, and lemon zest. Mix well. Arrange the thighs on a baking tray, and gently peel back the skin, leaving it attached.
2. Brush the thigh meat with a couple of teaspoons of the butter mixture and replace the skin to cover the meat.

Season with pepper. Bake for 40 minutes, until the skin is crisp, and the juices run clear. Let rest for 5 minutes before serving.

Serves: 6   Prep Time: 10 mins.   Cook Time: 40 mins.

Calories: 626; Fat: 17g; Carbs: 1g; Protein: 16g; Phosphorus: 114mg; Potassium: 158mg; Sodium: 120mg

Snacks
Deliciously Good Tuna Dip

Stage 3: Moderate damage in kidneys (eGFR = 30–59 mL)

Stage 4: Severe damage in kidneys (eGFR = 15–29 mL)

Ingredients:

- 1 can (170 g) no salt added tuna in water, drained
- 1 tsp lemon juice
- 1/2 tsp Dijon mustard
- 2 Tbsp light mayonnaise
- pepper to taste

Directions:

1. Place tuna in a bowl and shred. Add remaining ingredients and mix well. Best served with your low salt cracker or sourdough bread.

Serves: 4   Prep Time: 8 mins.   Cook Time: 0 mins.

Calories: 580; Carbs: 2g; Protein: 12g; Fat: 4g; Phosphorus: 76mg; Potassium: 140mg; Sodium: 86mg

Day 16

Breakfast

Buckwheat Pancakes

Stage 3: Moderate damage in kidneys (eGFR = 30–59 mL)

Stage 4: Severe damage in kidneys (eGFR = 15–29 mL)

Ingredients:

- 1¾ cups Homemade Rice Milk or unsweetened store-bought rice milk
- 2 teaspoons white vinegar
- 1 cup buckwheat flour
- ½ cup all-purpose flour
- 1 tablespoon sugar
- 2 teaspoons Phosphorus-Free Baking Powder
- 1 large egg
- 1 teaspoon vanilla extract
- 2 tablespoons butter, for the skillet

Directions:

1. In a small bowl, combine the rice milk and vinegar. Let sit for 5 minutes. Meanwhile, in a large bowl, mix the buckwheat flour and all-purpose flour. Add the sugar and baking powder, stirring to blend.
2. Add the egg and vanilla to the rice milk and stir to blend. Combine your dry and wet ingredients then stir. In a large

skillet over medium heat, melt 1½ teaspoons of butter. Use a ¼-cup measuring cup to measure the batter into the skillet.

3. Cook for 2 to 3 minutes; ensure that at the surface of the pancakes small bubbles form. Flip for 1 to 2 minutes till it cooks on the opposite sides. Transfer the pancakes to a serving platter, and in batches, continue cooking the remaining batter in the skillet, adding more butter as needed.

Serves: 4   Prep Time: 10 mins.   Cook Time: 15 mins.

Calories: 664; Total Fat: 9g; Carbs: 39g; Protein: 7g; Phosphorus: 147mg; Potassium: 399mg; Sodium: 232mg

Lunch

Bulgur and Broccoli Salad

Stage 3: Moderate damage in kidneys (eGFR = 30–59 mL)

Stage 4: Severe damage in kidneys (eGFR = 15–29 mL)

Ingredients:

- 3 cups broccoli florets
- 1 cup bulgur
- ½ cup cherry tomatoes, halved
- ¼ cup raw sunflower seeds
- ¼ cup chopped mint leaves
- Juice of 1 lemon
- 1 tablespoon extra-virgin olive oil
-

Directions:

1. In a medium bowl, prepare an ice-water bath by filling the bowl with ice and water. Set a pot of water on to boil. Add the broccoli and blanch for 3 minutes. With a slotted spoon,

remove the broccoli and transfer it to the ice bath, retaining the cooking water over the heat.

2. Once cool, after about 3 minutes, drain the ice and water. Set the broccoli aside. Add the bulgur to the hot water, remove from the heat, cover, and let sit for 15 minutes.

3. Drain, pressing the bulgur with the back of a spoon to remove excess moisture. In a medium bowl, toss the broccoli, bulgur, tomatoes, sunflower seeds, mint, lemon juice, and olive oil. Serve immediately.

Serves: 4   Prep Time: 10 mins.   Cook Time: 15 mins.

Calories: 456; Fat: 6g; Carbs: 24g; Protein: 6g; Phosphorus: 101mg; Potassium: 315mg; Sodium: 21mg

Dinner

Swiss Chard, White Bean & Pasta Soup

Stage 3: Moderate damage in kidneys (eGFR = 30–59 mL)
Stage 4: Severe damage in kidneys (eGFR = 15–29 mL)

Ingredients:

- ¾ cup fine egg noodles, cooked and drained
- 1 cup chopped canned tomatoes
- cannellini beans, 1 cup, dried
- red Swiss chard, 1 small bunch, stems removed, leaves julienned
- 1 tbsp olive oil
- 2 medium carrots, peeled and coarsely chopped
- 2 medium yellow onions, coarsely chopped
- 3 garlic cloves, minced
- 3 tbsp. finely chopped fresh basil
- 4 tbsp. finely chopped fresh flat leaf parsley

- 6 cups chicken broth
- 6 tbsp. Grated Parmigiano-Reggiano Cheese
- Pepper and sea salt to taste

Directions:

1. The night before, pick and discard any misshapen beans. Then soak while fully covered in water overnight. The next day, drain and discard water from beans. On medium high fire, place a soup pot and heat oil.
2. Add onions and sauté for 5 minutes or until soft. Add carrots, for 3 minutes, sauté it. Add half of Swiss chard and sauté for 3 minutes or until wilted. Add garlic, basil, tomatoes, beans and broth.
3. Simmer for an hour until beans are soft while partially covered. Turn off fire and with an immersion blender, puree soup until smooth. Turn on fire to medium high and add remaining chard and pasta.
4. Cook for 3 minutes. Season to taste with pepper and salt. Add 2 tbsp. parsley, mix well and turn off fire. To serve, ladle soup equally into serving bowls, garnish with remaining parsley and cheese.

Serves: 6   Prep Time: 15 mins.   Cook Time: 20 mins.

Calories: 531; Carbs: 30g; Protein: 13g; Fat: 7.3g; Phosphorus: 208mg; Potassium: 741mg; Sodium: 526mg

Snacks

Choco-Chip Cookies with Walnuts and Oatmeal

Stage 3: Moderate damage in kidneys (eGFR = 30–59 mL)

Stage 4: Severe damage in kidneys (eGFR = 15–29 mL)

Ingredients:

- ½ cup all-purpose flour
- ½ cup chopped walnuts
- ½ cup whole wheat pastry flour
- ½ tsp baking soda
- 1 cup semisweet Choco chip
- 1 large egg
- 1 large egg white
- 1 tbsp vanilla extract
- 1 tsp ground cinnamon
- 2 cups rolled oats (not quick-cooking)
- 2/3 cup granulated sugar
- 2/3 cup packed light brown sugar
- 4 tbsps cold unsalted butter, cut into pieces

Directions:

1. Position two racks in the middle of the oven, leaving at least a 3-inch space in between them. Preheat oven to 350oF and grease baking sheets with cooking spray.
2. In medium bowl, whisk together baking soda, cinnamon, whole wheat flour, all-purpose flour and oats. In a large bowl, with a mixer beat butter until well combined. Add brown sugar and granulated sugar, mixing continuously until creamy.
3. Mix in vanilla, egg white and egg and beat for a minute. Cup by cup mix in the dry ingredients until well incorporated.

85

Fold in walnuts and Choco chips. Get a tablespoon full of the batter and roll with your moistened hands into a ball.

4. Evenly place balls into prepped baking sheets at least 2-inches apart. Pop in the oven and bake for 16 minutes. Ten minutes into baking time, switch pans from top to bottom and bottom to top. Continue baking for 6 more minutes.

5. Remove from oven, cool on a wire rack. Allow pans to cool completely before adding the next batch of cookies to be baked. Cookies can be stored for up to 2-weeks in a tightly sealed container or longer in the ref.

Serves: 48   Prep Time: 20 mins.   Cook Time: 32 mins.

Calories: 471; Carbs: 12g; Protein: 2g; Fat: 3g; Phosphorus: 47mg; Potassium: 56mg; Sodium: 18mg

Day 17

Breakfast

Cereal with Cranberry-Orange Twist

Stage 3: Moderate damage in kidneys (eGFR = 30–59 mL)

Stage 4: Severe damage in kidneys (eGFR = 15–29 mL)

Ingredients:
- 1/4 cup dried cranberries
- 1/3 cup oat bran
- ½ cup orange juice
- ½ cup water

Directions:

1. In a bowl, combine all ingredients. For about 2 minutes, microwave the bowl then serve with sugar and milk. You may also add honey. Enjoy!

Serves: 1   Prep Time: 8 mins.   Cook Time: 5 mins.

Calories: 471; Carbs: 44g; Protein: 7g; Fat: 3g; Phosphorus: 249mg; Potassium: 406mg; Sodium: 7mg

Lunch

Lasagna Rolls in Marinara Sauce

Stage 3: Moderate damage in kidneys (eGFR = 30–59 mL)

Stage 4: Severe damage in kidneys (eGFR = 15–29 mL)

Ingredients:

- ¼ tsp crushed red pepper
- ¼ tsp non-iodized salt
- ½ cup shredded mozzarella cheese
- ½ cups parmesan cheese, shredded
- 1 14-oz package tofu, cubed
- 1 25-oz can of low-sodium marinara sauce
- 1 tbsp extra virgin olive oil
- 12 whole wheat lasagna noodles
- 2 tbsp Kalamata olives, chopped
- 3 cloves minced garlic
- 3 cups spinach, chopped

Directions:

1. Put enough water on a large pot and cook the lasagna noodles according to package instructions. Drain, rinse and set aside until ready to use.
2. In a large skillet, sauté garlic over medium heat for 20 seconds. Add the tofu and spinach and cook until the spinach wilts. Transfer this mixture in a bowl and add parmesan olives, salt, red pepper and 2/3 cup of the marinara sauce.
3. In a pan, spread a cup of marinara sauce on the bottom. To make the rolls, spread your noodle then top with ¼ cup of your tofu filling. Tightly roll then place it on the pan with the marinara sauce. Do this procedure until all lasagna noodles are rolled.
4. Place the pan over high heat and bring to a simmer. Reduce the heat to medium and let it cook for three more minutes. Sprinkle mozzarella cheese and let the cheese melt for two minutes. Serve hot.

Serves: 9   Prep Time: 15 mins.   Cook Time: 30 mins.

Calories: 600; Carbs: 65g; Protein: 36g; Fat: 26g; Phosphorus: 627mg; Potassium: 914mg; Sodium: 1194mg

Dinner

One-Pan Curried Chicken Thighs and Cauliflower

Stage 3: Moderate damage in kidneys (eGFR = 30–59 mL)

Stage 4: Severe damage in kidneys (eGFR = 15–29 mL)

Ingredients:

- 3 tablespoons curry powder
- ½ teaspoon ground cumin
- ¼ teaspoon paprika
- ½ teaspoon freshly ground black pepper, divided

- 6 bone-in chicken thighs
- 4 teaspoons extra-virgin olive oil, divided
- 1 cauliflower head, cut into florets
- ½ teaspoon dried oregano
- Juice of 2 limes

Directions:

1. In a small bowl, mix the curry powder, cumin, paprika, and ¼ teaspoon of pepper. In a medium bowl, drizzle 2 teaspoons of olive oil over the chicken thighs, and sprinkle with the curry mixture.
2. Cover, refrigerate, and marinate for at least 2 hours or up to overnight. Preheat the oven to 400°F. In a medium bowl, toss the cauliflower with the remaining 2 teaspoons of olive oil and the oregano.
3. In a single layer, arrange the chicken and cauliflower on a baking sheet. Bake for 40 minutes, stirring the cauliflower and flipping the chicken pieces once during cooking, until the chicken is well browned and its juices run clear. Drizzle with the lime juice and serve.
4.

Serves: 6   Prep Time: 10 mins.   Cook Time: 40 mins.

Calories: 575; Fat: 10g; Carbs: 8g; Protein: 16g; Phosphorus: 152mg; Potassium: 486mg; Sodium: 77mg

Snacks

Savory Collard Chips

Stage 3: Moderate damage in kidneys (eGFR = 30–59 mL)

Stage 4: Severe damage in kidneys (eGFR = 15–29 mL)

Ingredients:

- 1 bunch collard greens

- 1 teaspoon extra-virgin olive oil
- Juice of ½ lemon
- ½ teaspoon garlic powder
- ¼ teaspoon freshly ground black pepper

Directions:

1. Preheat the oven to 350°F. Line a baking sheet with parchment paper. Cut the collards into 2-by-2-inch squares and pat dry with paper towels. In a large bowl, toss the greens with the olive oil, lemon juice, garlic powder, and pepper. Use your hands to mix well, massaging the dressing into the greens until evenly coated.
2. Arrange the collards in a single layer on the baking sheet, and cook for 8 minutes. Flip the pieces and cook for an additional 8 minutes, until crisp. Remove from the oven, let cool, and store in an airtight container in a cool location for up to three days.

Serves: 4   Prep Time: 5 mins.   Cook Time: 20 mins.

Calories: 424; Fat: 1g; Carbs: 3g; Protein: 1g; Phosphorus: 6mg; Potassium: 72mg; Sodium: 8mg

Day 18

Breakfast

Blueberry-Oat Pancakes

Stage 3: Moderate damage in kidneys (eGFR = 30–59 mL)
Stage 4: Severe damage in kidneys (eGFR = 15–29 mL)

Ingredients:

- ½ cup + 2 tbsps agave nectar
- 1 cup frozen blueberries
- ½ cup Greek yogurt, vanilla flavor

- 1 cup milk
- 1 egg
- ½ tsp baking soda
- ½ tsp baking powder
- 1 cup whole wheat flour
- ½ cup steel cut oats
- 1 ½ cups water

Directions:

1. On high fire, add your water into a pot then set to boil. Add in your oats. Lower fire and allow to simmer for ten minutes or until oats are tender. Turn off fire and set aside.
2. Whisk egg in a medium bowl. Add yogurt and milk and whisk well. Sift in baking soda, baking powder and whole wheat pastry flour. Whisk well to combine. Fold in cooked oats and blueberries.
3. On medium fire, place a nonstick fry pan and grease with cooking spray. Pour ¼ cup of the batter into fry pan and cook for 2-3 minutes or until pancake is bubbly.
4. Turnover pancake and cook for a minute. Remove pancake and place in a serving plate. Repeat process for remaining batter until done. Serve and enjoy with your favorite syrup.

Serves: 10   Prep Time: 12 mins.   Cook Time: 1 hr.

Calories: 494; Carbs: 16g; Protein: 5g; Fat: 3g; Phosphorus: 144mg; Potassium: 165mg; Sodium: 19mg

Lunch

Bell Pepper 'n Garlic Medley on Sea Bass

Stage 3: Moderate damage in kidneys (eGFR = 30–59 mL)

Stage 4: Severe damage in kidneys (eGFR = 15–29 mL)

Ingredients:

- Bell Pepper, 1 Green, cored and chopped
- Bell Pepper, 1 Red, cored and chopped
- lemon, ½, juiced
- rice, 2–3 cups, cooked
- 3 Shallots, chopped
- 4 garlic cloves, minced
- Sea Bass, 4 skinless fillets (6-0z ea.)
- Private Reserve Greek extra virgin olive oil
- 1/2 tbsp ground coriander
- 1/2 tbsp garlic powder
- 1 tsp Aleppo pepper (or Sweet Spanish paprika)
- 1 tsp ground cumin
- 1/2 tsp black pepper

Directions:

1. In a small bowl, combine the last 5 ingredients to make the spice mixture. Set aside. In a medium-sized skillet, heat 2 tbsp olive oil over medium-high heat until hot, around 3 minutes.
2. Add the bell peppers, shallots, and garlic. Season with sea salt and preferred spices. Cook, while stirring, for 5 minutes until peppers are fork tender. Switch the heat to low.
3. Dry fish then season both sides with your spice mix. In a large cast iron skillet, heat 1/4 cup extra virgin olive oil over medium-high, around 7 minutes. Add fish pieces and push down on the middle (thickest part) for 30 seconds or so.
4. Allow your fish to cook for about 6 minutes on one side, flip and cook for 4 minutes on the other.
5. Switch off the heat, drizzle lemon juice. Serve hot with the bell pepper medley spooned on top. Enjoy!

Serves: 4   Prep Time: 18 mins.   Cook Time: 35 mins.

Calories: 543; Carbs: 37g; Protein: 34g; Fat: 16g; Phosphorus: 1273mg; Potassium: 1392mg; Sodium: 96mg

Dinner

Asian Chicken Satay

Stage 3: Moderate damage in kidneys (eGFR = 30–59 mL)

Stage 4: Severe damage in kidneys (eGFR = 15–29 mL)

Ingredients:
- Juice of 2 limes
- 2 tablespoons brown sugar
- 1 tablespoon minced garlic
- 2 teaspoons ground cumin
- 12 ounces boneless, skinless chicken breast, cut into 12 strips

Directions:
1. In a large bowl, stir together the lime juice, brown sugar, garlic, and cumin. Add the chicken strips to the bowl and marinate in the refrigerator for 1 hour. Heat the barbecue to medium-high.
2. Remove the chicken from the marinade and thread each strip onto wooden skewers that have been soaked in water. Grill the chicken for about 4 minutes per side or until the meat is cooked through but still juicy.

Serves: 6   Prep Time: 15 mins.   Cook Time: 10 mins.

Calories: 578; Fat: 2g; Carbs: 4g; Phosphorus: 116mg; Potassium: 208mg; Sodium: 100mg; Protein: 12g

Snacks

Walnut Butter on Cracker

Stage 3: Moderate damage in kidneys (eGFR = 30–59 mL)

Stage 4: Severe damage in kidneys (eGFR = 15–29 mL)

Ingredients:

- 1 tablespoon walnut butter
- 2 pieces Mary's gone crackers

Directions:

1. Spread ½ tablespoon of walnut butter per cracker and enjoy.

Serves: 1   Prep Time: 2 mins.   Cook Time: 0 mins.

Calories: 334; Carbs: 4g; Protein: 1g; Fat: 14g; Phosphorus: 19mg; Potassium: 11mg; Sodium: 138mg

Day 19

Breakfast

Summer Vegetable Omelet

Stage 3: Moderate damage in kidneys (eGFR = 30–59 mL)
Stage 4: Severe damage in kidneys (eGFR = 15–29 mL)

Ingredients:

- 4 egg whites
- 1 egg
- 2 tablespoons chopped fresh parsley
- 2 tablespoons water
- Olive oil spray, for greasing the skillet
- ½ cup chopped and boiled red bell pepper
- ¼ cup chopped scallion, both green and white parts
- Freshly ground black pepper

Directions:

1. In a small bowl, whisk together the egg whites, egg, parsley, and water until well blended; set aside. Generously spray a large nonstick skillet with olive oil spray and place it over medium-high heat.
2. Sauté the peppers and scallion for about 3 minutes or until softened. Add in your egg mixture then cook, swirling the skillet, for about 2 minutes or until the edges of the egg start to set.
3. Lift up the set edges and tilt the pan to allow even cooking. Continue lifting and cooking the egg for about 4 minutes or until the omelet is set.
4. Loosen the omelet with a spatula and fold it in half. Cut the folded omelet into 3 portions and transfer the omelets to serving plates. Season with black pepper and serve.

Serves: 3   Prep Time: 15 mins.   Cook Time: 10 mins.

Calories: 477; Fat: 3g; Carbs: 2g; Phosphorus: 67mg; Potassium: 194mg; Sodium: 229mg; Protein: 12g

Lunch

Mixed Green Leaf and Citrus Salad

Stage 3: Moderate damage in kidneys (eGFR = 30–59 mL)

Stage 4: Severe damage in kidneys (eGFR = 15–29 mL)

Ingredients:

- 4 cups mixed salad greens
- ¼ cup pepitas
- Juice of 1 lemon
- 2 teaspoons extra-virgin olive oil
- Freshly ground black pepper
- 1 orange, peeled and thinly sliced
- ½ lemon, peeled and thinly sliced
- 4 tablespoons (¼ cup) dried cranberries
- 4 tablespoons (¼ cup) pitted Kalamata olives

Directions:

In a large bowl, toss the greens, pepitas, lemon juice, and olive oil. Season with pepper.

Arrange the greens on four plates, and top each with 2 slices of orange and lemon. Add 1 tablespoon each of cranberries and Kalamata olives to each plate. Serve.

Serves: 4   Prep Time: 10 mins.   Cook Time: 0 mins.

Calories: 542; Fat: 9g; Carbs: 15g; Protein: 3g; Phosphorus: 116mg; Potassium: 219mg; Sodium: 137mg

Dinner
Asian-Style Pan-Fried Chicken

Stage 3: Moderate damage in kidneys (eGFR = 30–59 mL)

Stage 4: Severe damage in kidneys (eGFR = 15–29 mL)

Ingredients:

- 12 ounces boneless, skinless chicken thighs, fat removed, cut into 2 or 3 pieces each
- 1 teaspoon low-sodium soy sauce

- 1 teaspoon dry rice wine
- 1-inch piece ginger, minced
- ½ cup cornstarch
- 3 teaspoons canola oil, divided
- 1 lemon, cut into wedges

Directions:

1. In a medium bowl, combine the chicken, soy sauce, rice wine, and ginger. Toss and let sit for 15 minutes. Toss the chicken again and drain the liquid from the bowl. One at a time, dip the chicken pieces in the cornstarch to coat.
2. Set a half of your oil in a skillet on medium heat. Add half of the chicken to the pan and cook for about 3 to 5 minutes or until golden brown on one side. Flip, and continue to cook on the opposite side, until the chicken is cooked through and is golden brown.
3. Transfer the chicken to a plate lined with paper towels to cool. Repeat the process until done. Serve garnished with lemon wedges.

Serves: 4   Prep Time: 20 mins.   Cook Time: 25 mins.

Calories: 698; Fat: 7g; Carbs: 16g; Protein: 17g; Phosphorus: 148mg; Potassium: 218mg; Sodium: 119mg

Snacks

Roasted Mint Carrots

Stage 3: Moderate damage in kidneys (eGFR = 30–59 mL)

Stage 4: Severe damage in kidneys (eGFR = 15–29 mL)

Ingredients:

- 1 pound carrots, trimmed
- 1 tablespoon extra-virgin olive oil
- Freshly ground black pepper
- ¼ cup thinly sliced mint

Directions:

Preheat the oven to 425°F. Arrange the carrots in a single layer on a rimmed baking sheet. Drizzle with the olive oil, and shake the carrots on the sheet to coat. Season with pepper. Roast for 20 minutes, or until tender and browned, stirring twice while cooking. Sprinkle with the mint and serve.

Serves: 6   Prep Time: 5 mins.   Cook Time: 20 mins.

Calories: 451; Fat: 2g; Carbs: 7g; Protein: 1g; Phosphorus: 26mg; Potassium: 242mg; Sodium: 52mg

Day 20

Breakfast
Garden Salad with Strawberries

Stage 3: Moderate damage in kidneys (eGFR = 30–59 mL)

Stage 4: Severe damage in kidneys (eGFR = 15–29 mL)

Ingredients:

- ¼ cup red bell pepper, chopped
- ½ cup toasted pecans
- 1 cup sliced fresh strawberries
- ½ red onion, sliced
- 1 head romaine lettuce, torn into bite-size pieces
- 1 tbsp poppy seeds
- 1/8 cup distilled white vinegar
- ¼ cup white sugar
- ¼ cup milk
- ½ cup fat free creamy salad dressing

Directions:

1. Whisk well poppy seeds, vinegar, milk, and salad dressing in a small bowl. In a large salad bowl, mmix red bell pepper, pecans, strawberries, onion and lettuce. Pour in dressing, toss to coat well. Serve immediately.

Serves: 6   Prep Time: 10 mins.   Cook Time: 10 mins.

Calories: 540; Carbs: 14g; Protein: 4g; Fat: 10g; Phosphorus: 106mg; Potassium: 402mg; Sodium: 212mg

Lunch

Creamy Gorgonzola Polenta with Summer Squash Sauté

Stage 3: Moderate damage in kidneys (eGFR = 30–59 mL)

Stage 4: Severe damage in kidneys (eGFR = 15–29 mL)

Ingredients:

- ¼ cup fresh basil, chopped
- ½ tsp ground pepper
- ¾ cup cornmeal
- 1 14-oz cans of vegetable broth, divided
- 1 cup water
- 1 cup water
- 2 small yellow summer squash, sliced
- 2 small zucchinis, sliced
- 2 tbsp extra virgin olive oil
- 2 tbsp flour
- 2/3 cup crumbled Gorgonzola cheese
- 3 tbsp minced garlic

Directions:

1. In a saucepan, mix 2 ½ cups of broth and 1 cup water and bring to a boil under medium high heat. Reduce the heat to low once the liquid boils and cover the saucepan.
2. Stir occasionally until the mixture becomes thick and grainy. This should take 10 or 15 minutes. Once the mixture has

achieved a thick mixture, add the Gorgonzola cheese and remove from heat.
3. In a skillet, heat oil over medium high heat and add garlic. Sauté for 30 minutes and add the squash and zucchini and cook for five minutes.
4. Sprinkle the flour over the vegetables and add the remaining 1 cup of broth. Allow to boil then switch to low heat. Cook for three minutes.
5. Add the basil and serve the sauté over the polenta. Serve warm.

Serves: 4   Prep Time: 15 mins.   Cook Time: 50 mins.

Calories: 484; Carbs: 36g; Protein: 11g; Fat: 12g; Phosphorus: 187mg; Potassium: 333mg; Sodium: 438mg

Dinner
Squash and Eggplant Casserole

Stage 3: Moderate damage in kidneys (eGFR = 30–59 mL)

Stage 4: Severe damage in kidneys (eGFR = 15–29 mL)

Ingredients:

Vegetable:
- Pepper to taste
- 2 cups low sodium vegetable broth
- ½ cup dry white wine
- 1 red bell pepper, seeded and cut to julienned strips
- 1 eggplant, halved and cut to 1-inch slices
- 1 small butternut squash, cut into 1-inch slices
- 12 baby corn
- 1 large onion, cut into wedges
- 1 tbsp olive oil

Polenta:
- 2 tbsp fresh oregano, chopped
- ¼ cup parmesan cheese, grated
- 1 cup instant polenta

Topping:
- 5 tbsp parsley, chopped
- Grated zest of 1 lemon
- 1 garlic clove, chopped
- 2 tbsp slivered almonds

Directions:

1. Preheat the oven to 350 degrees Fahrenheit. In a casserole, heat the oil and add the onion wedges and baby corn. Sauté over medium high heat for five minutes. Stir occasionally to prevent the onions and baby corn from sticking at the bottom of the pan.

2. Add the butternut squash to the casserole and toss the vegetables. Add the eggplants and the red pepper. Cover the vegetables and cook over low to medium heat. Cook for about ten minutes before adding the wine. Let the wine sizzle before stirring in the broth. Bring to a boil and cook in the oven for 30 minutes.

3. While the casserole is cooking inside the oven, make the topping by spreading the slivered almonds on a baking tray and toasting under the grill until they are lightly browned. Place the toasted almonds in a small bowl and mix the remaining ingredients for the toppings.

4. Prepare the polenta. In a large saucepan, bring 3 cups of water to boil over high heat. Add the polenta and continue whisking until it absorbs all the water. Reduce the heat to medium until the polenta is thick. Add the parmesan cheese and oregano. Serve the polenta on plates and add the casserole on top. Sprinkle the toppings on top.

Serves: 8   Prep Time: 15 mins.   Cook Time: 1 hr.

Calories: 526; Carbs: 15g; Protein: 6g; Fat:5 g; Phosphorus: 117mg; Potassium: 618mg; Sodium: 222mg

Snacks

Cinnamon Apple Chips

Stage 3: Moderate damage in kidneys (eGFR = 30–59 mL)

Stage 4: Severe damage in kidneys (eGFR = 15–29 mL)

Ingredients:

- 4 apples
- 1 teaspoon ground cinnamon

Directions:

1. Preheat the oven to 200°F. Line a baking sheet with parchment paper. Core the apples and cut into ⅛-inch slices. Toss your cinnamon and apple slices to coat. Spread the apples in a single layer on the prepared baking sheet. Cook for 2 to 3 hours, until the apples are dry. They will still be soft while hot, but will crisp once completely cooled. Store in an airtight container for up to four days.

Serves: 4   Prep Time: 5 mins.   Cook Time: 3 hrs.

Calories: 596; Fat: 0g; Carbs: 26g; Protein: 1g; Phosphorus: 0mg; Potassium: 198mg; Sodium: 2mg

Day 21

Breakfast

Green Breakfast Soup

Stage 5: Kidney failure/End-stage CKD (GFR < 15 mL)

Ingredients:

- 2 cups spinach
- 1 avocado, halved
- 2 cups low-sodium vegetable or chicken broth (see Lower sodium tip)
- 1 teaspoon ground coriander
- 1 teaspoon ground cumin
- 1 teaspoon ground turmeric
- Freshly ground black pepper

Directions:

1. In a blender or food processor, add the spinach, avocado, broth, coriander, cumin, and turmeric. Process until smooth.
2. Transfer the mixture to a small saucepan over medium heat, and cook until heated through, 2 to 3 minutes. Season with pepper.

Serves: 2   Prep Time: 5 mins.   Cook Time: 5 mins.

Calories: 421; Fat: 18g; Carbs: 15g; Protein: 5g; Phosphorus: 58mg; Potassium: 551mg; Sodium: 170mg

Lunch

Cucumber and Radish Salad

Stage 5: Kidney failure/End-stage CKD (GFR < 15 mL

Ingredients:

- 2 large cucumbers, peeled and sliced
- 1 bunch radishes, sliced
- ½ sweet onion, sliced
- ¼ cup apple cider vinegar
- 1 tablespoon extra-virgin olive oil
- Freshly ground black pepper

Directions:

1. In a medium bowl, toss the cucumbers, radishes, and onion. Add the apple cider vinegar and olive oil and toss to coat. Season with pepper.

Serves: 6   Prep Time: 10 mins.   Cook Time: 0 mins.

Calories: 469; Fat: 4g; Carbs: 8g; Protein: 2g; Phosphorus: 52mg; Potassium: 386mg; Sodium: 29mg

Dinner

Chicken, Pasta, and Broccoli Bake

Stage 5: Kidney failure/End-stage CKD (GFR < 15 mL)
Ingredients:

- 8 ounces egg noodles

- 1 (10-ounce) package broccoli florets
- 2 tablespoons butter
- ½ sweet onion, chopped
- ¼ cup all-purpose flour
- 1½ cups Simple Chicken Broth or low-sodium store-bought chicken stock
- Freshly ground black pepper
- ¾ cup Homemade Rice Milk or unsweetened store-bought rice milk
- 3 cups shredded cooked chicken breast
- ¼ cup shredded Cheddar cheese

Directions:

1. Preheat the oven to 350°F. Grease a 2-quart baking dish. Set your water on in a pot ans allow to boil. Add the egg noodles and cook for 5 minutes. Add the broccoli and continue to cook for 3 to 5 more minutes, until the noodles are tender, and the broccoli is just fork-tender. Drain and set aside.
2. Set your butter on to melt in a medium saucepan over medium-high heat, heat the butter. Add the onion and cook for 3 to 5 minutes, until it begins to soften. Add the flour and stir until evenly mixed.
3. Add the broth and season with pepper. Simmer for 5 minutes, until it begins to thicken. Add the rice milk and cook until heated through. Toss the sauce with the broccoli, noodles, and cooked chicken, and transfer to the prepared baking dish. Top with the Cheddar cheese. Bake for 20 minutes, uncovered, until browned and bubbly.

Serves: 6   Prep Time: 15 mins.   Cook Time: 30 mins.

Calories: 651; Fat: 11g; Carbs: 38g; Protein: 24g; Phosphorus: 271mg; Potassium: 402mg; Sodium: 152mg

Snacks

Roasted Bananas with Chocolate Yogurt Cream

Stage 5: Kidney failure/End-stage CKD (GFR < 15 mL)

Ingredients:

- ½ cup whipping cream
- ½ tsp ground cinnamon
- 1 ½ cups low fat vanilla yogurt, chilled and drained
- 1 tbsp cold butter
- 1 tbsp confectioner's sugar
- 1 tbsp dark rum or lemon juice
- 2 tbsp unsweetened cocoa powder
- 3 tbsp dark brown sugar
- 4 bananas cut in strips

Directions:

1. Place bananas cut side up on a baking sheet coated with cooking spray. Sprinkle with brown sugar, rum and cinnamon. Dot with butter. Roast in a 425-degree Fahrenheit preheated oven for five minutes. Turn the broiler off until the bananas are golden.

2. Meanwhile, beat the cocoa, cream and confectioner's sugar in a large bowl using an electric mixer. Add the drained yogurt and fold the cream until well combined. Plate the roasted bananas and add a dollop of chocolate cream on top.

Serves: 4   Prep Time: 10 mins.   Cook Time: 5 mins.

Calories: 536; Carbs: 42g; Protein: 7g; Fat: 7g; Phosphorus: 186mg; Potassium: 727mg; Sodium: 91mg

Chapter 2: Shopping list

This section outlines some of the top super foods that you may want to consider incorporating into your diet. Depending on the stage of kidney disease you are at, certain foods may not be suitable for you. Please always check with your doctor or dietitian before adding or removing foods from your diet.

RED BELL PEPPERS: Red bell peppers are ideal for those suffering from chronic kidney disease as they are full of fiber, folic acid, vitamin B6, vitamin C and vitamin A while also being low in potassium. Another benefit for the kidneys is the high concentration of lycopene - an antioxidant that will increase kidney performance. Red bell peppers taste great in chicken or tuna salads or simply eaten with a low sodium dip. Roasted, they make a great addition to any salad or sandwich. They also add a mild kick to kebabs, egg dishes or as a part of a ground turkey or beef meal.

CABBAGE: Cabbage contains high amounts of phytochemicals which break down toxins, improve cardiovascular health and fight cancer. What's more, cabbage is a great source of folic acid, B6, fiber, vitamin C and vitamin K while still being low in potassium. Cabbage is a great addition to fish tacos or coleslaw and can be microwaved, steamed or boiled depending.

CAULIFLOWER: Cauliflower contains numerous compounds that help the liver to remove toxins from the body; it is high in fiber, folate, and vitamin C. Cauliflower is delicious with a simple dip, in salads, boiled or steamed. Cauliflower can be a great substitute for things like rice and potatoes and can be flavored using herbs, spices, and mustard.

GARLIC: Garlic is great used to replace salt for flavoring and seasoning and it also naturally lowers cholesterol and mitigates inflation. Garlic has fewer anti-inflammatory and anti-clotting effects once it has been cooked so is best consumed raw for maximum results.

ONION: Raw onions are low in potassium and high in chromium which is beneficial when it comes to helping the metabolism maintain its proper function. They can be consumed cooked or raw.

APPLES: High in fiber and vitamin content which helps to mitigate inflammation, apples have been linked to decreasing cancer risk, preventing heart disease, easing constipation and lowering cholesterol. They are just as healthy cooked as raw, and can also be consumed as a juice. Those who have been advised to restrict their water intake should avoid apples because of their significant water content.

CRANBERRIES: Cranberries are very acidic and help to prevent harmful bacteria from forming in the bladder, thus preventing infections in the urinary tract. They are also vitamin rich which can help to reduce the risk of heart disease or cancer. Cranberries are just as healthy when dried as they are when fresh and can be added to most salads or cereals for a delicious twist. Cranberry juice should be avoided for those on a restricted liquid intake.

BLUEBERRIES: High in antioxidants, fiber and vitamin C, blueberries also help to mitigate inflammation. Their manganese content helps prevent bone related issues that may occur as a result of a calcium deficiency. Blueberries can be eaten raw, dried, baked, in a smoothie, or with cereal.

RASPBERRIES: Also high in antioxidants, these little superfoods are known to help reduce cancer cells or tumor growth.

STRAWBERRIES: High in fiber, manganese, vitamin C and other vitamins and minerals which are known to help prevent cancer, maintain heart health and mitigate inflammation.

CHERRIES: Eating cherries daily has been shown to measurably reduce the amount of inflammation that those experiencing chronic kidney disease experience. They are also high in antioxidants as well as phytochemicals which help reduce the risk of heart disease. Cherries are great on their own, in desserts and also as a sauce for either pork or lamb.

RED GRAPES: Red grapes get their color from flavonoids which help to maintain heart health, reduce the risk of blood clots and improve oxidation and overall blood flow. They are also known to help reduce the risk of cancer and ease inflammation. Choose grapes the most vibrant in color. Frozen grapes taste delicious and are also thirst quenching, which is great if you are having to control your water intake.

EGG WHITES: Egg whites are pure protein; they are also lower in phosphorus than egg yolks, and they contain a wealth of vital amino acids. Egg whites can be eaten on their own, in salads, with tuna, or even in smoothies for those not on a liquid restricted diet.

FISH: Besides being a great source of protein, fish is known to be an anti-inflammatory agent thanks to its omega-3 content. Additional fats found in fish can help reduce the risk of heart disease as well as cancer. The healthiest fish in terms of omega-3 content are rainbow trout, herring, mackerel, tuna, albacore, and salmon.

OLIVE OIL: Olive oil has been linked to a reduced risk of both heart disease and cancer. Extra virgin olive oil contains higher levels of antioxidants than regular olive oil, making it a great choice for cooking, as a dip, marinade or dressing.

KALE: Loaded with flavonoids and carotenoids, both of which can reduce the risk of heart disease and cancer, kale is also full of calcium, vitamin C, vitamin A and vitamin K. Kale is a great snack choice as it can be baked and consumed as a chip.

VITAMINS & SUPPLEMENTS: Vitamins and supplements that you would usually buy in shops should be avoided when on a renal diet as they may contain high levels that cannot be regulated by the kidneys anymore. Your healthcare professional may prescribe you a vitamin suitable for kidney disease patients, so please consult with them first.

FOODS TO AVOID OR CUT DOWN

DAIRY: It is sometimes advised to limit your consumption of dairy whilst on a renal diet, this will help monitor your protein intake as well as control the amount of fat you eat. Try swapping full-fat cheddar and parmesan for cottage cheese or brie.

CAFFEINE: Caffeine is a stimulant which is hard for the kidneys to filter. Moreover, consuming caffeine on an empty stomach has been linked to the formation of kidney stones and can also lead to an increase in calcium levels found in the urine. Try reducing the amount of caffeine you drink slowly; this will prevent withdrawal symptoms and ensure healthier functioning kidneys for longer. Green tea is a great caffeine-free alternative to coffee and tea but it boosts energy in the same way as caffeine does, making you feel great.

ARTIFICIAL SWEETENER: Avoid artificial sweeteners like saccharin and opt for Stevia if you need something to sweeten up your teas or meals.

SODA: Soda is harmful to both your kidneys as well as your bones, in fact, drinking just 32 oz. of soda per day is known to measurably increase your risk of chronic kidney disease. Avoid soda on a kidney-friendly diet.

GMO's: Genetically modified organisms are likely to increase the number of free radicals present in foods; the chemicals and toxins in these foods cannot be filtered by the kidneys properly.

POTATOES: Sweet potatoes and white potatoes are high in potassium and should be monitored. They can be leached by soaking them in warm water or boiling twice prior to cooking to remove excess potassium. Sweet potatoes come with many other vitamins and minerals so it is important to consult your doctor or dietitian to find out whether you can include potatoes in your diet and what quantities.

TOMATOES: Tomatoes are also high in potassium. Canned tomatoes with no added salt or sugar can be consumed in moderation. Please consult your doctor or dietitian to find out whether you need to avoid tomatoes completely.

TIPS FOR EATING OUT:

Firstly, don't be embarrassed to make specific requests when eating out. Your health is more important than seeming to make a fuss and most of the time servers will be more than happy to meet your needs. If not, they're not worth your custom!

- Always ask for vegetables and side salads to be served plain and cooked dry without oil or butter.
- Avoid deep-fried and breadcrumbed foods as these are often cooked in huge quantities of bad oils.
- When choosing steak, ask or opt for a smaller cut and have sides of vegetables, salads or suitable grains to fill you up.
- Seafood, chicken, and turkey are better options but ensure they're baked, poached, steamed or boiled. If shallow fried, ask for them to cook this in olive oil.
- Try smaller or half portions if you're going to have a starter and a main.
- Ask for olive oils or vinegar on the side so you can control the amount you put on your food.
- Limit your alcohol intake and order a small glass. Ask waiters and waitresses not to top this up if you're somewhere fancy!
- Print the list of foods above or perhaps keep it electronically on your phone so you can easily check food types and opt for the best choice when dining out.

If visiting friends and family members, share this list with them so they can make the best choices for everyone and not worry about whether they are doing the right thing.

RENAL DISEASE AND THE DIET

Consult your doctor as often as you can: the kidneys are your body toxin's filter, and you should always try to clean your blood from toxins and preservatives in food.

Try not to eat irresponsibly (foods, drinks and even the air you breath) as many elements can be turned into something bad like formaldehyde due to a chemical reaction and morphing phase, which can lead to renal failure, cancer or various other problems.

Renal failure happens when your kidneys are not able to get rid of toxins and wastes in your blood, and this is called chronic kidney disease" or "chronic renal failure."

This is a progressive problem, and it can be found out, treated, the diet changed, and it might also be possible to resolve what is the cause of the problem. It usually takes a long time to get to renal failure and you certainly to want to reach it because this would require dialysis treatments to save your life, to clean the blood and remove the toxins in the blood using a machine because your body can no longer do this job. Without treatments, you could die a very painful death. It can be the result of long periods of high blood pressure, irresponsible diet, diabetes.

The renal diet uses a low quantity of proteins and phosphorus, sodium, and this will control the toxins in your blood, helping your kidneys functions. If you adjust your diet very fast and early, you could prevent total renal failure.

THE RENAL DIET FOR DIABETIC PATIENTS

For diabetics who suffer from renal disease, there is a specific diet known as diabetic renal diet. Very often, this diet is also conceived for diabetics who want to avoid incurring in renal diseases.

114

Diabetics and patients with renal disease often have problems in eating the right food.

The aim of this diet is to have glucose levels within the right range. This is possible by not missing any meals, by having a regular diet, by eating low glycemic carbohydrates, in order to help the body always have the same level of glucose and low glycemic foods are grains bread, sweet potatoes, and brown rice. However, if the diet is for renal problems, you should also avoid sweet potatoes and grain bread, as they are rich in potassium.

People with renal problems, as we have already seen, should avoid food rich in potassium phosphorus and sodium. Since sodium is often present, patients should look carefully at labels, and dietitians should advise patients to avoid sodas with dark colors, coffee, and drinks with too much sodium for diabetics with renal problems.

Unsweetened teas, water, and clear diet sodas are allowed. As for vegetables, broccoli, cauliflowers, beets, eggplant, and cabbage are recommended for their vitamin-rich features, together with their low potassium and carbohydrates content. You should then avoid meat such as sausage, bacon, and organ meats.

Also, avoid canned vegetables as they are rich in sodium: nutritionists will also guide you on portion sizes to help your blood glucose control.

Many people suffering from renal problems also have diabetes. The main goal for diabetic diets is to maintain the right level of glucose in your blood. This can be done by:

- Eating carbohydrates with a low glycemic index (GI) such as grains, unrefined foods, most fruits and vegetables, legumes, sweet potatoes (only in some quantities), nuts.

- White bread, sugar, confectionaries, drinks with added sugar should be avoided

- Eating small frequent meals is a good habit. Don't go long periods without eating and don't do huge meals or even worse, do not skip meals.

The renal diet then tries not to stress kidneys, and this can be done by:

- Limiting daily intake of proteins: an excess of proteins need to be broken into carbohydrates and nitrites which, in the form of urea, can be destroyed by urine as it causes stress on already damaged kidneys.

- Limiting table salt and do not use a salt replacement as they contain potassium.

- Reduce also potassium and phosphates, including apricots, avocado, bananas, kiwi, watermelon, peaches, prunes as phosphorus avoid legumes, dairy products, dried legumes, shellfish, organ meats.

The renal diet for diabetics food pyramid:

This is a pyramid (divided into 5 groups) which indicates appropriate eating, where the larger group is made up of grains, rice, beans, starchy vegetables.

Then we have a smaller group including fruits and vegetables

A smaller quantity is dedicated to food with less fat and salt. If you drink alcohol, take it in moderate quantities. Choose food high in fibers and vitamins and minerals, such as whole grain and be physically active at least 30 minutes a day.

Eat frequently with small and repeated meals, when you wake up in the morning eat your first meal and then every 2-3 hours, taking your last meal at bedtime.

PLEASE NOTE:

If you plan your full week it will be easier for you to follow the diet, always fill up the plate with half of it with vegetables and salads, then the other half with proteins or carbohydrates.

No salt, and instead of it use fresh herbs, spices, onions, garlic, lemon juice.

For smaller meals eat whole grain cereals, crackers or bread, fruit, a glass of skim milk, nuts, yogurt, plenty of salads, or a small quantity of cottage cheese.

This diet can be powerful in both controlling renal failure and diabetes. Stick to your diet, and you will feel better and healthier.

HOW TO MANAGE DIABETES AND RENAL DISEASES EFFECTIVELY

Diabetic renal diet is a subject of interest as diabetes mellitus is one of the most common extrarenal diseases affecting the kidneys.

Diabetes mellitus leads to diabetic nephropathy in 30% of cases and to its end stage.

The diabetic renal diet is conceived to help metabolic control in these types of patients. By controlling diabetes mellitus, we can also control the worsening situation of kidneys and prevent end-stage renal disease.

The kidney metabolizes 30-40% of insulin, and as the renal functions decline, the degradation of insulin also decreases, leading to a lower insulin need. Renal failure can be identified when the patient is evaluated for recurrent insulin reactions.

Renal disease can be controlled by

- checking hypertension carefully
- adjusting insulin therapy
- restricting protein in your diet.

However, renal failure appears within 5 to 10 years after the first appear of proteinuria (protein in urine).

The following are some recommendations for patients with diabetes mellitus.

- total calories: to maintain reasonable weight in adults, meet increased needs in children, adolescents, pregnant and lactating women and people recovering from catabolic illness
- caloric distribution: 50 to 70 % of carbohydrates, 20 to 30% of proteins, 20 to 30% of fats
- cholesterol limited under 300mg/day or less
- sodium below 300mg/day less for people with hypertension and renal complications
- alcohol: a very moderate amount
- vitamin and mineral supplements: to be given to individuals with low caloric diets (1200 kcal/day)

The diet for an individual with diabetes can only be a dietary prescription based on nutrition assessment and treatment goals. The diabetic renal diet can be a good guideline to control and manage diabetes mellitus, which may then go into renal diseases.

Conclusion

A renal diet is an eating plan conceived to help people who suffer from renal diseases. It can expand the effectiveness of treatment by lowering the level of waste products in their blood.

This diet is designed to avoid stressing kidneys, and it provides useful nutrients and energy to the body.

The diet is based on some basic rules.

The main rule is that it must be a healthy and balanced diet, rich in fibers, natural grains, carbohydrates, omega 3 fats, vitamins and fluids. Protein should be present but not excessively, they are essential to rebuild tissues but cannot be exceeding in this diet as excessive quantities of proteins should be broken down by the body into carbohydrates and nitrates. Moreover, as nitrates are not used by the body, they should be excreted through the kidneys.

Salts are kept to a minimum and electrolyte levels of blood are checked on a regular basis and are then balanced accordingly. Please inform your doctor before starting the diet.

Carbohydrates are important for energy and need to be taken in the right quantities. However, you should avoid refined ones. You should try to use as many whole grains and unrefined forms of carbohydrates as possible.

Table salt should be used only for cooking and remember that excessive salt causes retention and stress to the kidneys. Salty foods should be avoided as well: no sausages, no snacks, no tinned food.

There is also the level of phosphorus which needs to be monitored carefully, avoiding colored drinks like colas and food with a high level of potassium such as bananas, citrus fruits, apricots, dark leafy green vegetables should be avoided too, especially if blood levels rise.

Take into consideration also Omega 3 fats which are important in your diet but avoid trans-fats and hydrolyzed fats.

The proper renal diet can really help kidneys functioning longer, and it has only more restrictions on proteins and table salt, while restrictions to phosphorous and potassium can be needed if the levels of blood rise and the signs of accumulation become too evident.

Part 2

The structure of the kidney

The kidneys are two paired organs located on either side of the spine at about the level of the lower ribs.

Every healthy kidney is about 9 to 12 cm long, 4 to 6 cm wide and 3 to 5 cm thick, depending on the size of the human body. Together, the two kidneys weigh only about 300 g. The surface of healthy kidneys is usually smooth. Since they perform many tasks for the body, they are very well supplied with blood. About 1,800 liters of blood flow through the kidney daily.

In the renal cortex are many small blood vessel balls, the so-called glomeruli. In these glomeruli, the blood vessel wall is permeable to various components of the blood. While the blood cells, i.e. red and white blood cells, and plasma albumin (blood protein) cannot escape from the blood vessel, glucose (sugar), urea, electrolytes, and water pass through the vessel walls and are collected in the so-called tubules. The fluid collected in the tubules is called primary urine. Approx. 125 ml of primary urine are formed in this way every minute. This equates to almost 180 liters per day. The primary urine contains salts, nutrients, and slags, but no blood cells and no protein. Excretion via the kidneys is mainly ensured by two different mechanisms:

The tubules run meandering through the renal cortex and the medulla adjacent to the middle of the kidney. In this way, many components of the primary urine and almost all the fluid are reabsorbed and remain with the body. This leads to a concentration of the primary urine; the result is the actual urine (urine). This contains, in a healthy kidney daily, about 20 to 30 g of urea, 0.25 to 0.75 g of uric acid, 0.5 to 1.8 g of creatinine and 0.7 to 1.5 g of phosphate.

In the body, the kidneys are responsible for:
- fluid and electrolyte balance
- the regulation of blood pressure
- detoxification, as well as regulation of urea and creatinine

- the regulation of the acid-base household
- the regulation of red blood cell formation as well
- the production of hormones and enzymes

Chronic kidney disease usually progresses slowly. With the help of blood and urine examinations, it is possible to estimate whether the kidneys are still working adequately or, for example, dialysis should be started soon.

Blood and urine tests are not only necessary to detect chronic kidney disease. Also, in the further course, regular controls are very important: They show if and if so, how fast the illness progresses and help to estimate the risk of complications. Depending on the stage of the disease, the therapy can be adapted individually, and the next treatment steps can be discussed and planned in good time with the doctor. This is important, for example, when it is foreseeable that dialysis will be necessary.

Chronic kidney failure

Chronic renal failure (renal insufficiency) causes a deterioration of renal function. This increases the concentration of urinary substances in the blood (substances that have to be eliminated via the kidneys), e.g. creatinine and urea. The regulation of the water, electrolyte and acid-base balance is impaired. After the kidney forms hormones or activates vitamins, it can, among other things, lead to disorders of blood formation and changes in bone metabolism.

The kidneys can be damaged by inflammatory processes, vascular changes and various other diseases (high blood pressure, diabetes mellitus, and genetic factors). Chronic kidney disease develops over months or years; usually, both kidneys are affected.

Which stages can the disease go through?

Chronic kidney disease is divided into five stages:

Stage 1: Urinalysis shows signs of kidney damage. Healthy areas of the kidneys, however, ensure that they still function as normal.

Stage 2: In addition to kidney damage, kidney function is also slightly limited. Usually, however, no symptoms are noticeable.

Stage 3: Kidney function is moderately limited.

Stage 4: Kidney function is severely limited. There may already be episodes such as itching, anemia, hyperacidity or bone pain.

Stage 5: Terminal Renal Failure: The kidneys can no longer sufficiently cleanse the blood - there is often pronounced uremia. A dialysis or kidney transplant is needed to restore kidney function.

The health consequences of chronic kidney disease also depend on the state of health. Therefore, doctors are also investigating what could accelerate the progression of kidney failures - such as heart disease, a poorly adjusted high blood pressure or diabetes mellitus.

This is important to adapt the medication therapy individually - or to plan further steps with sufficient lead: For example, if you have a high risk that your kidneys will fail in the foreseeable future, you can discuss the treatment with the doctor as soon as possible. Perhaps more close follow-up examinations will be necessary.

What are the causes of chronic kidney failure?

The triggers for chronic renal failure are mainly various diseases in question, for example:

Diabetes Mellitus: This is responsible for 40 per cent of all cases of chronic renal failure (diabetic nephropathy). High blood glucose levels in the long term damage the walls of the blood vessels and the other filter structures in the kidneys, making them more permeable to small protein particles, especially albumin. These are increasingly excreted in the urine. Also, a decline in filter particles (glomeruli) leads to a progressive reduction in detoxification performance.

Inflammation of the filter particles in the renal corpuscles (glomerulonephritis, but also systemic diseases such as lupus erythematosus): Approximately every fourth chronic renal insufficiency is caused among other things by immune and autoimmune reactions, infectious diseases or tumors.

Cystic kidney and other genetic disorders: This congenital malformation causes about eight percent of all cases of chronic renal failure. The kidney function is restricted, e.g. by fluid-filled cavities (cysts).

Hypertension: Increased blood pressure damages the glomeruli and blood vessels in the kidney over time. Paradoxically, in kidney disease increased blood pressure, more hormones are formed and less fluid is excreted. Impaired kidney function and hypertensive condition mutually reinforce each other.

Diseases of the blood vessels, e.g. atherosclerosis: may lead to reduced renal blood flow.

Medicines: The kidneys filter drugs and their breakdown products from the blood. Some substances can damage the kidney tissue, e.g. certain antibiotics, analgesics, and cytostatics.

What symptoms can occur?

Chronic kidney disease is often insidious and causes very different symptoms depending on the stage of the disease. In the beginning, there are usually no or only slight complaints. Only in case of a rapid deterioration of renal function can the first signs of illness already occur, e.g.:

- increased excretion of light urine,
- High blood pressure,
- Edema in the legs, but also other parts of the body (e.g. eyelids),
- Red-colored urine (through the blood), foaming urine (through protein admixture).
- Greater renal impairment may, among other things, cause the following symptoms:

- Symptoms of anemia, such as skin blanching, feeling cold, tiredness, weakness,
- Concentration and memory disorders,
- decreasing physical capacity,
- Nausea,
- Vomiting,
- Diarrhea,
- Itching and burning in the legs,
- Muscle and bone pain.

In the advanced stage, almost all organ systems are impaired by the lack of detoxification function of the kidneys. Typical end-stage symptoms (terminal kidney failure) include:
- Non-adjustable hypertension,
- The decrease in the amount of urine,
- Water retention
- Shortness of breath,
- Nausea,
- Vomiting,
- loss of appetite,
- irregular heartbeat,
- Drowsiness, drowsiness,
- Cramps,
- Coma.

Main causes & risk factors

Common causes of chronic kidney failure are diabetes mellitus and high blood pressure, which account for about 35% of all cases. 15% of renal insufficiency patients suffer from inflammatory diseases of the renal corpuscles, the so-called glomerulonephritis. Hereditary diseases such as cystic kidney (8%) and kidney-damaging drugs or chronic renal pelvic inflammatory disease (5% each) are other causes. The various diseases lead to different rates of decline in kidney function.

Blood sugar and blood pressure significantly influence the development and progression of chronic renal failure. Even a slight increase in blood pressure can speed kidney weakness along with diabetes. The systolic pressure in healthy people is in the range of 110-130 mmHg, the diastolic pressure is 70-80 mmHg. A pressure of 140/90 and above is considered elevated blood pressure.

However, the reasons for chronic kidney failure are not always known. There seems to be a genetic predisposition, as people with kidney-related relatives are also more likely to get kidney disease. In addition, we know today that obesity and smoking can increase the risk of chronic kidney failure.

Diabetes

The common cause of chronic kidney failure is diabetes. If the blood sugar level increases for a long time, there is a risk of chronic kidney disease. Increased blood sugar permanently damages the walls of the blood vessels. This hinders the blood flow and thus the nutrient transport to the organs. The late damage of diabetes in the kidneys is called diabetic nephropathy.

By damaging the small blood vessels in the kidneys, their wall becomes more permeable. Small protein particles, called albumins, slip through the vessel walls and are excreted in the urine. The detection of albumin in the urine is the first warning sign that diabetes causes damage to the kidneys. The narrowing of the small blood vessels in the kidneys also means that the kidney tissue is no longer sufficiently supplied with oxygen and nutrients, and the kidney cells die off.

Glomerulonephritis

The renal corpuscles are the "microfilters" of the kidneys and are also called glomeruli, which consist of tiny, coiled-up blood vessels that filter salts, metabolites, pollutants and, most importantly, fluid from the blood. Each kidney has about half to one million glomeruli contaminants in the blood that can cause the cells of the kidneys to become inflamed. Inflammations always affect both kidneys and, more or less, all kidney bodies.

Polycystic kidney disease

This congenital renal malformation usually leads to renal insufficiency from the age of 40 years. Numerous fluid-filled cavities (cysts) restrict the function of kidney tissue. In childhood, these cysts are small, fill up more and more in the course of life with fluid and then displace the normal kidney tissue. This leads to renal insufficiency, which often leads to dialysis in the sixth decade of life.

High blood pressure

High blood pressure can both be the cause and consequence of chronic kidney weakness. On the one hand, high blood pressure damages the kidney bodies (glomeruli), so that they gradually fail. On the other hand, with decreasing renal function increased blood pressure, increasing hormones are formed. In addition, there is too much salt and water in the body, which also raises blood pressure.

Impaired kidney function and high blood pressure condition and reinforce each other. In many cases, hypertensive patients are, therefore, also kidney patients at the same time and vice versa.

Drugs

As an important excretory organ of the body, the kidneys also filter many drugs or their degradation products. However, some of these substances can damage kidney tissue. Medication-related kidney damage is generally rare and can occur only at very high doses (e.g. acetaminophen, see below) or in patients with certain risks. Medications that can occasionally cause such kidney damage include:

- Painkillers, such as paracetamol, ibuprofen, diclofenac
- Antibiotics, such as B. aminoglycosides (amikacin, gentamycin, neomycin or streptomycin)
- Anticancer drugs (chemotherapeutics)
- Iodinated contrast media

Over-the-counter painkillers can cause kidney damage if taken for long periods. Thus, the active ingredient paracetamol from a total dose of 1,000 grams has a kidney-damaging effect - an amount that is achieved with the twice-daily intake of 500-milligram tablets after three years. Also, in the long-term use of pantoprazole and other blockers of gastric acid (so-called PPIs), kidney damage is increasingly being discussed recently.

Improper use or wrong dosage of even hypertension and diuretic drugs (diuretics) may trigger a more acute renal failure.

Diseases of the blood vessels

Chronic diseases of the blood vessels can impair kidney function. Vascular diseases can lead to reduced blood flow and thus trigger reduced blood flow to the kidneys. If there are deposits of lime and fats (so-called plaques) on the vessel wall, as is the case with arteriosclerosis, the vessels can gradually close completely, so that the underlying kidney tissue is no longer supplied with blood and dies. This can also affect blood vessels that are outside the kidneys. For example, if there is a constriction between the abdominal aorta and the kidney, this is called renal artery stenosis.

Blood vessels can also become inflamed; this is called vasculitis (from the Latin vas for blood vessel). Such vasculitis sometimes occurs only at the kidney, more often the kidney and other organs are affected. They often run very fast, i.e. kidney function can be completely lost within weeks. Fortunately, the doctors have very good medicines to cure vascular inflammation, at least in case of a timely diagnosis.

Chronic kidney weakness: first signs & symptoms

First signs

The beginning of a chronic kidney weakness is often marked only by low signs of disease or even runs completely symptom-free. Often the kidney problems are superimposed by the symptoms of the underlying disease, such as the symptoms of diabetes or vasculitis.

Early symptoms of kidney disease can be:
- Increased excretion of less colored, light urine
- Increased blood pressure
- Water retention (edema) on the legs, around the eyes or all over the body
- Red urine

Symptoms

A gradual course with little or no discomfort is characteristic of chronic renal insufficiency. An initially occurring high blood pressure of over 140/90 mmHg or an increasingly difficult to set high blood pressure can be an early sign of disease.

Many patients often produce bright, low-concentration urine and store water in the skin and subcutaneous tissue (edema). Foaming urine when urinating may be an indication of protein in the urine. A healthy kidney excretes at most 200 milligrams of protein per day, of which at most 30 milligrams of the blood protein albumin. At higher values, one speaks of microalbuminuria, starting from 300 milligrams albumin per day of proteinuria. Some patients also excrete blood with the urine. If this occurs in larger quantities, the urine is colored red (gross hematuria). Most of the time, however, there is only so little blood in the urine that it is invisible to the naked eye and can only be recognized by test strips (microhematuria).

With the progressive loss of function, the kidneys can no longer fulfill their tasks. It comes to disturbances of the water balance, the acid-base and the electrolyte balance and other organ systems. Also, the body is more susceptible to infections. Since the kidneys no longer produce sufficient amounts of the hematopoietic hormone erythropoietin (EPO), the number of red blood cells decreases. Such anemia leads to fatigue, weakness, difficulty concentrating and decreasing exercise capacity.

A noticeable paleness of the skin is another possible clinical indication. Besides, patients often experience nausea, vomiting, or diarrhea shortly before starting dialysis. Other symptoms may include memory impairment, itching and burning in the legs and muscle and bone pain.

In the advanced stage of chronic renal failure, almost all organ systems are damaged by the lack of detoxification function of the kidneys (uremic syndrome). There are abnormal changes in the cardiovascular system, the hematopoietic system, the gastrointestinal tract, the peripheral and central nervous system, the skin, the hormone system, and the bones.

Typical symptoms of end-stage renal failure (terminal kidney failure) are:

- Unacceptable high blood pressure
- Decrease in urine output
- Water retention (edema)
- shortness of breath
- Nausea, vomiting, loss of appetite
- Irregular heartbeat
- Drowsiness
- Convulsions, coma

With the help of the so-called Glomerular Filtration Rate (GFR), chronic renal insufficiency is divided into five stages. The GFR is a laboratory value that is 90-130 milliliters per minute for normally functioning kidneys. This means that a healthy kidney purifies at least 90 milliliters of blood from freely filterable substances per minute and excretes them via the urine.

Stage I: GFR greater than 90 milliliters/ minute

Patients often have no symptoms at this stage. The blood levels for creatinine are still normal, only the protein excretion via the urine may be increased, or there are other indications, for example, as in the ultrasound, a kidney disease. If possible causes are already recognized, a worsening of the disease can very often still be prevented.

Stage II: GFR between 60-89 milliliters/ minute

Even at this stage, the kidney weakness is often not yet seen by blood tests. The kidneys still seem to function adequately, but more detailed studies show kidney disease, for example, with the measurement of urine protein or ultrasound. In addition, more accurate measurements, such as creatinine clearance, can detect a beginning of kidney failure.

Stage III: GFR between 30-59 milliliters/ minute

Renal damage has now progressed so fast that elevated creatinine and urea levels are also measured in the blood. Those affected suffer from high blood pressure, reduced performance, and faster fatigue. In stage III, the risk of cardiovascular disease increases significantly. The symptoms allow for different interpretations and do not necessarily indicate kidney weakness. Medicines that are normally excreted through the kidneys must now be reduced in their dose, so they do not cause any side effects.

Stage IV: GFR between 15-29 milliliters/ minute

At this stage, so many kidney cells are already defective that the deficient elimination of toxins affects the entire organism. The symptoms, therefore, increase the loss of appetite, tiredness, vomiting, nausea, nerve pain, itching, and bone pain. Because the body excretes fewer salts and water, it also leads to edema.

Stage V: GFR below 15 milliliters/ minute

If the kidney function is severely limited or the kidneys are eliminated, it is also called end-stage renal failure. The blood must be regularly cleaned at this stage by a blood wash (dialysis) of toxins. Otherwise, the body is poisoned. In spite of regular blood lavage, terminal renal insufficiency may still result in a yellowish discoloration of the skin and itching of the skin. Both are due to the deposition of substances in the skin, which would have to be excreted via the urine.

Kidney weakness (chronic): effects & complications

Disorders of blood purification, as well as the water and salt balance, affect many other organs of the body. Chronic renal insufficiency can, therefore, lead to various complications:

High blood pressure

An important consequence of a chronic renal failure is increased blood pressure: About 80% of the so-called kidney patients suffer from it. However, high blood pressure can also be the cause of kidney weakness. With decreasing urine output, the body cannot get rid of excess salt and water, which raises blood pressure. In addition, this leads to fluid retention, especially in the legs (edema). In extreme cases, fluid accumulates in the lungs, causing coughing with whitish to foamy secretions and severe shortness of breath (pulmonary edema).

Heart failure, cardiac arrhythmia, heart attack, stroke

In addition, there is further damage in the cardiovascular system, in particular to a pronounced calcification of arteries and also heart valves. Thus, valvular heart disease or heart failure occurs as a result of chronic kidney failure, and of course, heart attack and stroke through the calcified arteries. The kidneys increasingly lose the ability to regulate potassium in kidney failure, especially with a daily urine volume of less than one liter, the potassium levels in the blood can rise (hyperkalemia), which is characterized by a slowed heartbeat, dizziness and short loss of consciousness as well as muscle weakness and tingling sensations. Cardiac arrhythmias threaten cardiac arrest in greatly increased potassium levels. The excess water can also lead to a heart attack or stroke.

Disorders of the nervous system

Neurological disorders are also a common complication of advanced chronic renal failure. They can be measured as slowed nerve conduction velocity and altered brain waves in the electroencephalogram (EEG).

Possible symptoms are:

- Fatigue, memory and concentration disorders
- Optical hallucinations, disorientation, coma
- Itching, burning, muscle cramps or muscle weakness
- cognitive disorders
- sleep disorders
- anemia

As kidney function weakens, lower levels of the hematopoietic hormone erythropoietin are also produced. This leads to anemia, the so-called renal anemia, which can manifest itself through increased fatigue, a striking pallor of the skin and declining physical resilience.

Disorders of bone metabolism

As renal function decreases, less active vitamin D is available to the body. Active vitamin D is a hormone that promotes the absorption of calcium via the intestine and the strength of the bones. If in the kidney, too little active vitamin D is formed, then the calcium content in the bone decreases, there are more fractures and more bone, muscle and joint pain. In addition, since the damaged kidneys excrete less phosphate, the phosphate level in the blood increases, which additionally promotes decalcification of the bones and the calcification of the arteries.

High phosphate levels in the blood cause itching, bone pain, and muscle aches. In addition, the increased accumulation in the body increases the risk of arteriosclerosis. This increases the risk of heart attack and stroke.

Malnutrition

Disturbances in protein and energy metabolism, hormonal imbalances, as well as nausea and loss of appetite are the reasons why many kidney disease patients are malnourished, especially when protein metabolism is affected. Thus, the body absorbs fewer proteins with decreasing kidney function, and thus the calorie intake can go down.

Pregnancy & kidney weakness

Chronic kidney failure is more likely to result in premature birth, death of the unborn child, or birth defects. Complications of the mother may include bleeding, coagulation disorders, and hypertension. The risk, however, varies individually. Pregnant women with kidney disease must, therefore, be cared for by experienced doctors.

If the creatinine level in the blood is significantly increased, a viable child is rarely born. In normal creatinine, the higher the amount of protein in the urine, the more problematic the pregnancy. In about 5-10% of first-time mothers, urine protein is increased towards the end of pregnancy. A combination of increased urinary protein increases blood pressure and water retention in the tissue (edema), this is called gestosis.

Water retention can occur in any pregnancy. This explains a lot of the weight gain. After delivery, this fluid is excreted again, and the mother loses the extra body weight. Sometimes, however, stronger edema accumulates. These are disturbing but not dangerous, as long as there is no protein in the urine, and the blood pressure remains normal. In this case, the doctor can treat the water retention with leg elevation, less salt consumption, and support stockings. On the other hand, diuretics should not be given during pregnancy as they can slow down the flow of blood to the mother cake.

Kidney weakness (chronic): examinations & diagnosis

Many kidney diseases lead to long-lasting, irreversible kidney tissue damage. In contrast to acute renal failure, timely treatment can, in most cases, lead to stabilization or even recovery of renal function. The medical history of the patient and the physical examination play an important role.

For his diagnosis, the doctor must know about pre-existing kidney damage, chronic illnesses, and taking medications. Also, evidence of kidney disease in the family of the person affected is important.

The measurement of blood pressure and heart rate as well as the condition of the skin and the filling of the jugular veins allow conclusions on the fluid balance and thus on a possible water overload. With a 24-hour blood pressure measurement, the doctor can determine whether a patient has a normal blood pressure during the day, but suffers from unnoticed nocturnal hypertension. This is common in diabetics. Lack of nocturnal drop in blood pressure significantly increases the risk of organ damage.

By means of an ultrasound examination, the kidney size and the condition of the kidney tissue can be determined. If the kidneys are very small, this is an indication of long-standing kidney damage.

Blood test

When the kidneys are unable to filter the blood adequately, creatine and urea accumulate in the blood. The doctor can control this by analyzing blood levels. The more creatinine and urea in the blood, the weaker the kidney filter function. The creatinine normal is 8-12 milligrams per liter of blood, the normal urea concentration in the blood between 200 and 450 milligrams per liter. As an alternative to creatinine, cystatin C in the blood is measured as the control value, but so far, this is not yet a routine examination.

The concentration of creatinine in the blood is used in routine clinical practice for a preliminary assessment of renal function. However, this is not very accurate for all people, as the creatinine level often increases only when renal function has dropped by almost half. Thus, a slight restriction of kidney function can be overlooked.

More suitable for an early diagnosis is the so-called creatinine clearance, which indicates how quickly the kidneys can filter out creatinine from the blood. For this, urine must be collected for 24 hours and creatinine in the blood and urine is determined at the same time. Reduced creatinine clearance is found before the rise of creatinine in the blood and can, therefore, early indicate damage to the kidneys. In addition, the physician calculates the glomerular filtration rate from creatinine in blood serum or another small substance in the blood, cystatin C.

In addition, the doctor will determine the number of white blood cells and other blood levels, such as C-reactive protein, liver values , and fat levels. The C-reactive protein is increasingly produced during inflammatory processes in the liver and can indicate the course of renal insufficiency. Along with the blood picture, which has increased white blood cells in inflammatory processes, can be found next to the medical history, evidence of inflammation in the body.

The measurement of calcium, phosphate, vitamins and parathyroid hormone provides information about a disturbed electrolyte balance and possible damage to the bones.

Urinalysis

Since there is usually little or no protein in the urine, urinary excretion of protein is an important indicator of the presence of kidney disease. For this purpose, the urine is collected and analyzed for over 24 hours. Alternatively, the physician can determine the ratio of protein to creatinine in the urine. In a healthy kidney, the filter tissue is so dense that no more than 200 milligrams of protein per day is excreted in the urine. Regular measurements of protein excretion are also an important part of monitoring disease progression, as more and more protein is detected in the urine as the disease progresses.

A rapid urine test with a test strip allows the doctor to make an initial assessment of kidney disease. The test strips measure the protein content and the blood cells in the urine. If the test result is conspicuous, the urine must be further tested for the type and amount of these proteins and cells.

The so-called glomerular filtration rate (GFR) is another laboratory value by which the doctor can detect chronic urinary weakness early in the urine. With their help, he can assess the severity of the disease. The normal value of the glomerular filtration rate for creatinine is 90-130 milliliters per minute. That is, a healthy kidney purifies at least 90 milliliters of blood per minute.

In a microscopic examination of the urine, the so-called urine sediment, the doctor looks for red and white blood cells. If there is evidence of damage to the renal corpuscles, it may be necessary to perform a puncture of the kidney for tissue collection and examination.

Chronic renal insufficiency: treatment

Untreated chronic renal insufficiency often leads after years to a complete failure of the kidneys (terminal kidney insufficiency), in particular with hereditary diseases of the kidneys or if much protein is present in the urine. The more treatment can reduce protein levels in the blood, the sooner it can prevent complete kidney failure.

The goal of any treatment is to prevent or at least delay the progression of the disease. Complete healing is not possible in most cases, but the sooner kidney failure is treated, the better the chances of success. In some hereditary diseases such as the familial cystic kidney, however, there is still no therapy.

One differentiates between the treatment of the disease, which is based on kidney weakness, such as diabetes, hypertension or glomerulonephritis, as well as asymptomatic treatment, which should mitigate the effects of renal insufficiency, such as anemia, edema, potassium increase. The early treatment of the underlying disease is a prerequisite for the successful treatment of renal insufficiency.

If kidney failure is not yet very advanced, it can be treated with medication. Later, usually, an artificial blood purification (dialysis) or kidney transplantation is required.

Medication
- Diabetes medications

In diabetes mellitus, blood-sugar-lowering drugs, antihypertensive agents for high blood pressure and anti-inflammatory drugs are used for inflammation of the renal corpuscles. A good blood sugar and blood pressure control and permanent control of these two values can prevent kidney disease from occurring in the first place or slow down the progression of existing kidney failure.

- Blood pressure medications

In hypertensive patients, antihypertensive agents may slow the progression of diminishing renal function. In this case, so-called ACE inhibitors and angiotensin II receptor antagonists are preferably used, which in addition to the blood pressure-lowering effect also hardly burden the kidneys. Significantly, the kidney-protective effect of ACE inhibitors is independent of blood pressure. Thus, the ACE inhibitors are also prescribed at normal blood pressure levels. The target value is a blood pressure of 130/80. To achieve this, in many cases, several drugs with different mechanisms of action must be used. Patients can support drug therapy through physical activity, not nicotine and low salt diet.

- Inflammation

Inflammation of the renal corpuscles (glomerulonephritis) can be treated with drugs that reduce the activity of the immune system. These so-called immunosuppressants include drugs, such as cortisone, cyclosporin or cyclophosphamide.

- Hormones

As renal insufficiency also reduces the formation of new red blood cells, in the case of anemia (renal anemia), the kidney hormone erythropoietin (Epo) is administered, which promotes blood formation and thus increases the number of red blood cells. Before using Epo, the doctor will measure the amount of iron in the body, as chronic kidney weakness and anemia often lack iron.

- Fat reducers

Blood lipid-lowering drugs, such as statins are used for the treatment of elevated cholesterol levels and the treatment of cardiovascular diseases such as arteriosclerosis.

- Diuretics and phosphate binders

Diuretic drugs, also known as diuretics, increase salt and water excretion. Although the drugs can increase the amount of urine, they do not improve the detoxification function of the kidneys. If a low-phosphate diet can no longer keep phosphate levels stable as the renal function progresses, so-called phosphate binders (calcium carbonate, potassium acetate, calcium citrate) are used. These bind some of the phosphates in the food already in the gastrointestinal tract. They should be taken in the correct dosage immediately before or at the beginning of the meal.

Treatment with vitamin D and/or vitamin D analogs also serves to normalize calcium and phosphate metabolism.

- Dialysis

According to current guidelines, the initiation of renal replacement therapy (dialysis) is recommended at the latest with a creatinine clearance of fewer than 5-10 milliliters/minute, in diabetes patients also earlier. If a patient is already suffering from damage to many organs (uremic syndrome), or if edema or high blood pressure can no longer be brought under control, kidney replacement therapy should also be started earlier.

The preparation and initiation of renal replacement therapy must be timely. An adequate nutritional status, a well-adjusted blood pressure, and a balanced blood count are important prerequisites.

If there is a terminal renal insufficiency despite all therapeutic measures, only dialysis or kidney transplant can help. This is the case when the consequences of impaired kidney function through an adapted diet and medication are no longer manageable. Since early-onset improves treatment prospects, preparations should begin in a good time. Today, there are two different blood purification methods: on the one hand hemodialysis as the most commonly used procedure and the other hand, peritoneal dialysis.

- Kidney transplant

In a kidney transplant, a kidney patient receives a healthy kidney from a living or deceased donor. The surgeon transplants the patient either a kidney from a dead or a living relative or close people. This is possible without health restrictions for the donor, because of the two kidneys, which each person usually owns. A single kidney is sufficient for blood purification and urine production.

The prerequisite for organ removal for a donation from a deceased person is the determination of brain death according to the German Transplantation Act, which came into force in 1997. In the case of a living donation, no economic motives or emotional constraints may influence the decision for the donation. The prerequisite is that the blood type and other specific genetic characteristics of donor and recipient match so that the recipient's immune system does not repel the new kidney.

Diet in renal insufficiency

Nutrition has a major impact on the treatment and disease course of kidney failure. Anyone who adheres to the recommendations of the doctors or dieticians, therefore, can significantly support the treatment of chronic renal insufficiency.

Acute renal insufficiency

Acute renal failure may lead to increased protein degradation and lipid metabolism disorders. Pay attention to your calorie intake. Recommended are 35 to 40 kilocalories per kilogram of body weight and day.

Drink about as much as you left the day before. If the urine excretion is too low, patients should eat potassium, sodium and low protein. If the urine excretion is too high, a potassium and sodium-rich diet are recommended. This compensates for the loss of mineral salts. You can eliminate fluid loss by drinking enough.

Chronic renal insufficiency

Chronic renal insufficiency: low protein diet

Reduced protein intake may appear to slow the progression of renal insufficiency. Therefore, you should not consume more than 0.6 to 0.8 grams of protein per kilogram of body weight per day.

The consumed protein should have a high biological value, i.e. consist of many protein building blocks, which the body cannot form itself (essential amino acids). The combination of different protein sources ensures the supply of all important compounds. Ideal protein mixtures include, for example, potato and egg, beans and egg, milk and wheat, egg and wheat, as well as legumes and wheat.

Also recommended is the use of low-protein specialty products such as low-protein flour and products made from it (bread, pastries).

Chronic renal insufficiency: a diet low in phosphate

Chronic renal insufficiency has negative effects on bone metabolism, among other factors - bone stability decreases. In order not to increase this effect even further, a low-phosphate kidney diet is recommended, because too much phosphate makes the bones more brittle.

The recommended amount of phosphate is 0.8 to 1 gram per day. Restrict the consumption of high-phosphate foods. These include, for example, nuts, cereals, offal, and wholemeal bread. Many dairy products such as milk, yoghurt, and buttermilk also supply a lot of phosphates. Cheaper cheeses such as cottage cheese, cream cheese, Camembert, Brie, Mozzarella, Harzer Roller and Limburger are cheaper.

If possible, avoid foods with production-related phosphate additives such as processed cheese, cooked cheese, canned milk, and some sausages. You may want to ask about the phosphate content when buying sausages in the butchery. On the ingredient list of foods, you can see phosphate additives on the E numbers E 338 to E 341, E 450 a to c, E 540, E 543 and E 544.

Incidentally, there is a close link between the phosphate and protein content - protein-rich foods usually also contain a lot of phosphates.

Chronic renal insufficiency: low potassium diet

Especially in the advanced stage of renal insufficiency, patients should eat low-potassium, so as not to increase the increased potassium due to renal insufficiency in the blood. Too much potassium can cause cardiac arrhythmias.

Depending on the severity of the kidney weakness, a potassium intake of 1.5 to 2 grams per day is recommended. The best way is to avoid potassium-rich foods and drinks. These include:

- Fruit and vegetable juices
- Dried fruit (raisins, dates, figs)
- nuts
- Bananas, apricots, avocado
- Pulses (peas, beans, lentils, etc.)
- Tomatoes, spinach, Swiss chard, broccoli, kale, Brussels sprouts, fennel, olives
- Sprouts and germs
- Mushrooms (fresh and dried)
- Potato dry products (potato chips, potato dumplings, and mashed potatoes)

Chronic renal insufficiency: the amount of drinking

Although many patients suspect the opposite: drinking a lot cannot improve kidney function. Rather, over-hydration can even accelerate the progression of chronic renal insufficiency. Talk to your doctor or dietician about how much fluids you should take daily.

Chronic renal insufficiency: diet on dialysis

Limited fluid intake is particularly important in patients whose chronic renal insufficiency necessitates dialysis treatment.

Keeping a limited amount of fluid requires a lot of discipline. The daily amount of drinking depends on the urine excretion within 24 hours. As much fluid as you excrete, you should also reintroduce the body - plus about half a liter extra per day. Keep in mind, however, that you can cover some of your fluid requirements through your diet. Not only soups, but almost all foods contain water (for example, fruits, vegetables, yogurt, pudding, fish, and meat).

Tips for thirst-quenching:

- Chewing gum without sugar
- Suck ice cubes
- Lemon pieces suck
- Avoid salty and very sweet foods
- Rinse mouth

People with renal insufficiency who are on dialysis should control their weight daily. If the weight gain exceeds the level recommended by the physician, you should consult your doctor immediately.

Non-allowed foods

To reduce sodium

- Broth nuts, meat extracts
- Foods in brine, in salt, in oil (capers, olives, meats or canned fish)
- Margarine, mayonnaise, mustard, other sauces
- Milk powder
- Savory snacks, peanuts, popcorn
- To reduce phosphorus
- Sausages in general and sliced meats
- Cheeses with the exception of ricotta and mozzarella
- Chocolate
- Brewer's yeast
- Offal (liver, kidney, heart, brain, etc.) and fatty meats: lamb, goose, duck, chicken, game.

144

- Egg yolk
- Dried vegetables
- Dried fruit
- Crayfish
- Flour
- Bran

To reduce potassium

The limitation of foods rich in potassium should be carried out only on the precise indication of the treating nephrologist, as many foods rich in potassium have important health values and can help prevent the onset of cardiovascular diseases so frequently associated with this disease.

- Grapefruit, bananas, chestnuts, coconuts, kiwi, dried fruit
- Fruit juices
- Artichokes and spinach
- Potatoes
- Bran
- Integral products
- Dietary salts
- legumes
- mushrooms
- Sausages
- Ham
- Soy
- Bitter cocoa and chocolate
- Milk powder
- Parsley
- Sardines, sardines, stockfish
- Brewer's yeast

FOODS ALLOWED WITH MODERATION

Salt: It is a good rule to reduce the amount added to the dishes during and after cooking and limit the consumption of foods that naturally contain high quantities (canned or brine foods, nuts, and meat extracts, soy-type sauces). Common salt should not be replaced with "dietary salts" because they are rich in potassium.

100 cc wine for lunch and 100 cc for dinner or 150 cc of beer for lunch and 150 cc for dinner, with the doctor's permission.

Coffee: Limit consumption, if the doctor does not completely forbid it, to two cups a day.

Honey, jam, and sugar: Although free of phosphorus, they must be consumed in moderation due to their simple sugar content.

To reduce sodium

- Pizza, bread, crackers, and breadsticks.
- To reduce phosphorus
- Milk, yogurt, cream
- Pasta, rice, barley
- Fresh legumes
- Chocolate
- Fish
- Fresh cheeses such as ricotta and mozzarella

Allowed and recommended foods

Pasta, pana, rice

Tuscan bread. Tuscan bread can be replaced with breadsticks without salt or rusks without salt

Aproteic foods specially produced without proteins, which can improve the palatability of the diet such as bread, pasta, rice, flour, crackers, rusks, biscuits, and allow more acceptable portions of dishes that contain animal proteins. These foods are also available in supermarkets.

Meat, all types except very fat ones. Choose the leanest and least veined parts. Poultry skin must be discarded.

Fish, fresh or frozen except for fat varieties. Fresh fish must be washed in plenty of running water because sometimes it is stored in water and salt or under ice and salt before selling.

Vegetables, both fresh and frozen, excluding legumes (beans, chickpeas, lentils, broad beans, peas). Mushrooms and artichokes can be eaten only occasionally.

Fruit, with the exception of the aforementioned one, can be consumed either fresh or cooked, in a fruit salad or pureed without the addition of milk.

Seasonings prefer the use of extra virgin olive oil or choose seed oil (not of various seeds but of a single seed, for example, corn oil, peanut oil, sunflower oil).

Natural or mineral water.

Spices and aromatic herbs

Behavioral advice

In the case of overweight or obesity, it is recommended to reduce the weight and the "waistline," which is the abdominal circumference, an indicator of the quantity of fat deposited on a visceral level. Waist circumference values greater than 94 cm in men and 80 cm in women are associated with a "moderate" cardiovascular risk, values greater than 102 cm in men and 88 cm in women are associated with a "high risk." Obesity is a cause of kidney failure.

Maintain an active lifestyle compatible with the degree of the illness (abandon sedentariness! Go to work on foot, by bicycle or park far away, if you can avoid the use of the elevator and take the stairs on foot)

Read the product labels, especially to ascertain their micronutrient content.

Adequate control of blood pressure. Maintain optimal blood pressure values by reducing the intake of salt and alcohol and/or using antihypertensive drugs.

Check body weight in the morning before breakfast. The increase of 1 kg of body weight or more in a short time (a few days), the appearance of swelling, or the reduction of diuresis, should not be underestimated, it should be referred to a specialist doctor.

If you are diabetic, check your blood sugar carefully.

Beware of drugs. Do not take anti-inflammatories without the advice of the nephrologist.

Not smoking. Smoking damages the kidneys.

Practical tips

To further reduce the amount of potassium in food, it is advisable to soak the vegetables and fruit in cold water 8-9 hours before consumption and boil them in abundant water.

To further reduce the amount of phosphorus in food, it is recommended to soak them in a container and keep them in the fridge 8-9 hours before cooking. Prefer cooking like boiling in plenty of water; it is also recommended to change it halfway through cooking

Simple nutrition tips

Less phosphorus

Phosphorus from food is absorbed in the intestine and excreted through the kidneys. If there is limited kidney function, this can lead to phosphate overload in the body. As a possible long-term consequence, particularly vascular calcifications, they must be feared. A low intake of phosphorus is hardly conceivable with a central European diet, as it is contained in many foods.

Particularly rich in phosphorus, for example, finished products, since the mineral is often part of a variety of additives. Melted cheese, for example, is one of the foods with extremely high phosphorus content due to its melting salts. One slice already covers a quarter of the maximum recommended amount in kidney failure. Meat, fish, eggs and dairy products should not be consumed in excessive quantities because of their content.

Phosphorus from plant sources such as whole-grain cereals, nuts or legumes is absorbed by the intestine to a much lesser extent and is, therefore, less of a problem.

Less sodium

Saline is the largest source of sodium in the western diet. The average Austrian usually eats about one third more saline than

148

recommended. Ingesting too much salt through food may cause high blood pressure, over-hydration and, subsequently, left heart hypertrophy in patients with renal insufficiency. Like phosphorus, salt hides in considerable quantities in finished products, munchies, processed meat products, and cheese. A frozen pizza, for example, covers on average, three-quarters of the daily recommended maximum amount of table salt. Therefore, as far as possible, do not use finished products and do not salt them at the table.

Balanced ratio

To optimally support the metabolism with reduced kidney function, it can help to select the main nutrients protein, fat, and carbohydrates. Although protein is an important component of the body cell, however, too much animal protein - as is common in the general Austrian diet - can lead to increased acidity in the body. Especially the high consumption of meat and sausage ensures that the average Austrian absorbs about one third more protein than recommended. On the one hand, the most important measure should be to pay attention to small portion sizes and, on the other hand, to limit the frequency of consumption of animal protein carriers such as meat, poultry, eggs, sausages, and dairy products.

Particularly favorable is the combination of increased vegetables and fewer animal proteins. From the age of 65, the protein intake can be slightly increased again, as protein synthesis decreases with increasing age. The amount of ingested fat can basically be based on the situation of the person concerned. Due to the high energy value, it should be used sparingly in case of overweight. On the other hand, with the risk of malnutrition, increased fat intake can contribute to a good nutritional status.

Still fed up

To compensate for the smaller portion of meat, sufferers can eat plenty of complex carbohydrates and fiber. Vegetables, lettuce and carbohydrate-rich side dishes such as potatoes, rice, and noodles cause good satiety and have no negative impact on kidney function. This also applies to diabetics, if it is paid attention to, it is good for controlling blood sugar.

The currently very popular carbohydrate-reduced diets, in which precisely those supplements for weight loss are avoided, usually provide automatically for increased protein intake. Therefore, they are not suitable for people with chronic renal failure. Every day two hands full of fruit and plenty of vegetables - no matter in which form - supplement the diet with filling and digestive fiber as well as vitamins and minerals.

Rethinking dialysis

Once chronic kidney disease has become so advanced that renal replacement therapy in the form of hemodialysis or peritoneal dialysis becomes necessary, some of the nutritional needs of patients change. For example, a higher protein intake benefits the patients, but often the consumption of fruits and vegetables has to be limited. By that time at the latest, a detailed nutritional consultation by a doctor or dietician should take place.

Dietary guidelines

The following are some essential dietary guidelines concerning proteins, potassium restriction, phosphorus restriction, sodium restriction, and moisture restriction.

Protein

Proteins (= proteins) are the building blocks of the body and have different functions. They are essential for building muscle, providing protection against infections, ensuring the repair and renewal of cells in our body. A balanced intake of proteins through the diet must be sought. How many proteins are allowed daily depends on the remaining kidney function (no kidney replacement therapy) or the type of kidney replacement therapy (hemodialysis or peritoneal dialysis).

Proteins are broken down to urea, are then released into the blood as waste and are usually excreted by the kidneys. Proteins are found in many foods, but not always in the same amount.

Meat, fish, cheese, eggs, dairy products, and soy contain high-quality proteins.

Bread, potatoes and grain products (rice, pasta, etc.) also contain proteins but to a lesser extent and of lesser quality, but these foods are indispensable as an energy source.

· If the kidneys function less well (= renal failure), but kidney replacement therapy is not yet required, it is essential that the protein intake through the diet does not rise too high.

The less well-functioning kidneys excrete fewer waste materials (including proteins). The proteins absorbed through the diet must be of good quality.

If kidney replacement therapy is already required, the daily protein intake through the diet is higher since dialysis causes an additional loss of protein. A protein deficiency would lead to muscle weakness, reduced resistance, malnutrition, etc. what should be prevented.

Phosphorus restriction

The terms phosphate and phosphorus are often used interchangeably. Phosphorus accumulates in the blood if the kidneys not or insufficiently excrete it. Too much phosphorus in the blood can lead to bone loss, joint pains and itching. During dialysis, part of the phosphorus is removed from the blood. Part of this will also be removed via phosphate-binding medication prescribed by the doctor. However, these measures are often not sufficient, so that the intake of phosphorus via the diet must also be limited. Phosphorus is mainly found in foods that contain proteins. Protein-rich foods are, therefore, even phosphorus-rich foods. In addition to a lot of salt, most types of cheese also include a lot of phosphorus and are not recommended for people with kidney disease. Phosphorus is also used as an additive to soft drinks, which also have no nutritional value so that they are avoidable. A good knowledge of which foods contain phosphorus and the correct use of phosphate binders is essential here. Some tips regarding the use of phosphate binders:

- Take the phosphate binders during meals. The phosphate binders then come together with the food in the intestines. In this way, most of the phosphorus from the protein-rich meals can be bound.
- Also consider the protein-rich snacks such as yogurt, pudding, and cheese that are phosphor-rich because phosphate binders may then also be required.
- If you do not eat, for example, during illness, then naturally phosphate binders should not be taken.

Phosphorus is mainly in the following foods:
- Whole grain products (wholemeal and brown bread, brown rice and pasta, muesli, whole grain breakfast cereals, dried fruit cereals)
- Meat, meat products, fish, meat substitutes, egg yolk
- Milk and milk products, cheese, cheese spread
- Certain types of vegetables: mainly artichoke, corn, mushrooms, and sprouts
- Certain types of fruit: dried fruit and passion fruit
- Products based on cocoa (chocolate, chocolate spread, cookies with chocolate, pralines, etc.)
- Nuts, seeds, seeds, legumes
- Cola, beer and lawyer

Potassium restriction

Potassium is an essential mineral and helps the heart to function properly. Usually, the kidneys regulate the amount of potassium in the body. With reduced kidney function, the excess potassium is not removed and accumulates. Too high a potassium level in the blood can cause serious cardiac arrhythmias. The level of potassium in your blood can be reduced by restricting the use of potassium-rich foods. Potassium is mainly found in the following foods:
- Potatoes

- Whole-grain cereals (whole-grain and brown bread, brown rice and pasta, muesli, whole-grain breakfast cereals, dried cereal breakfast cereals)
- Vegetables, fruit and dried fruit
- Milk and milk products
- Certain drinks (strong coffee, fresh or ready-to-buy fruit, and vegetable juices
- Cocoa-based products (chocolate, chocolate spread, chocolate cookies, pralines, etc.)
- Nuts, seeds, seeds, and legumes
- Dietary products without salt and substitute salt

Some facts and tips about potassium:

Potassium is soluble in water. When boiling vegetables and potatoes in plenty of water, about 1/3 of the potassium is lost if you discard the boiling water at the end of the boiling process and replace it with fresh boiling water (so-called "boiling in two times").

* Potatoes are particularly potassium-rich. Replacing the potatoes with white rice or white pasta a few times a week is a good habit. White rice and white pasta (spaghetti, spirelli, macaroni, tagliatelle, noodles, etc.) contain much less potassium compared to potatoes and are therefore good alternatives.

* When using vegetables rich in potassium, replace the portion of potatoes with a piece of white rice or white pasta.

* Coffee can be replaced by tea or soft drinks. These drinks hardly contain any potassium.

* Preparation method of potatoes and vegetables:

- Potatoes:

Always peel the potatoes, cut them into small pieces and boil them twice in water, throwing out the first boiling water. Finish with mash, baked potatoes, croquettes, etc. if necessary. Potatoes cooked in the peel lose practically no potassium and are therefore best avoided.

- Vegetables:

Clean the vegetables and cut them into small pieces. Boil the plants once in a generous amount of water. Then drain the cooking liquid. After all, there is a lot of potassium in this boiling fluid, and it should therefore not be used to prepare a sauce. Finish the greetings with a little fat if necessary.

* Avoid cooking in the microwave, in a steam device, in a pressure cooker or baking in the oven, wok. These cooking techniques can only be used to heat already cooked potatoes and vegetables.

Sodium restriction

Sodium is a mineral that occurs in the body and is indispensable for certain functions of the body, such as water management.

If the kidneys are still functioning normally, the excess of sodium will be discharged. If the kidneys no longer work optimally, too much sodium remains in the blood. Too much sodium in the blood and salt (= NaCl) in the diet leads to thirst, fluid retention and an increase in blood pressure.

Sodium is a natural component of salt (= NaCl). By salt, we mean table salt, sea salt, salt enriched with iodine,

If one is advised to use less salt (NaCl), then it is actually meant that one must limit the sodium through the diet. Sodium is naturally present in almost all foods. For example, potatoes and vegetables do not contain a small amount of sodium during the preparation without adding salt. For many foods, sodium is added extra during the production process in the factory.

Some tips on how to reduce salt intake:

- do not add extra salt when preparing the meal or at the table;

limit the use of foods that are high in salt, such as:

- Smoked fish and meat and imposed products;
- Cheese, processed cheese, melted cheese;
- Ready-made spice mixtures (e.g. for spaghetti, barbecue, salads), sauces, canned soups, instant soup;

- Ready-made (frozen and fresh) meals, breaded meals (fish steaks, schnitzel), prepared frozen vegetables (e.g. leeks in cream sauce);
- Seasonings, such as stock cubes, mustard, ketchup, soy sauce.
- Salty snacks such as salty peanuts, crisps, aperitif cookies, cheese.
- Solid cheeses and French cheeses contain more salt compared to cheeses such as flat cheeses, cottage cheese, mozzarella, ricotta, ...;
- use other flavorings instead of salt, such as fresh herbs, spices, onion, garlic, lemon, etc. An herbal guide can help with this.
- Finish a dish with a twist of the pepper mill;
- Meat and fish can be seasoned well in a marinade (without salt);
- Unprepared frozen foods (vegetables, meat, fish, etc.) do not contain any added salt;
- Always give preference to fresh products (vegetables, meat, fish, etc.);
- Sea salt and iodine-enriched salt contain as much sodium as common kitchen salt;
- Preferably use low-salt bread or unsalted rusks;
- If the bread itself is baked, add less salt;
- Prefer fish and meat preparations in papillote and roasting. The taste is better preserved.
- DO NOT use substitute salt or diet products with less salt (low-salt cheeses, low-salt meats).

Caution for "diet salt" or "replacement salt"

These products often contain less or no sea salt, but sodium is often replaced by potassium which is not suitable for a potassium restriction! Moreover, this way, you maintain poor habituation to the salty taste.

Humidity limitation

A certain amount of fluid is necessary for everyone since our body consists of approximately 2/3 of water. Normally, an excess of ingested fluid is removed by the kidneys. With impaired renal function, fluid accumulates in the body, resulting in fluid retention (edema), feeling tight and increased blood pressure. All these can be prevented provided that there is an adjusted (limited) fluid intake (individually). The amount of fluid that can still be used daily depends, among other things, on the remaining urine production and is calculated according to the amount of urine that is still formed in 24 hours.

The permitted drink per day = 500 ml to 750 ml PLUS the number of ml urine output in 24 hours

The drink includes not only water, but also coffee, tea, soft drinks, soup, milk, custard, sauce, fruit juice or vegetable juice, etc.

In addition, solid foods naturally also bring in a certain amount of moisture. For example, vegetables, fruit, and potatoes consist of 90% water.

The total amount of moisture that is added daily by the solid foods is approximately 500 ml. These are not included in the permitted amount of drink per day (500 ml to 750 ml). A few tips to better maintain

Your fluid restriction:

- spread your fluid intake throughout the day;
- Use small cups, small glasses, etc. to distribute the amount of moisture better;
- Drink with small nibs and prefer fresh, not too sweet drinks;
- At parties, it is best to choose drinks that are served in small quantities (sherry, (foam) wine, champagne, spirits such as whiskey, cognac, etc. but in moderation) instead of soft drinks, beers, cocktails, ...;
- To avoid feeling thirsty, it is best to avoid as many salt-rich, sugar-rich and highly spiced (spicy) foods as possible;
- Take your medication with the meal or dessert (e.g. pudding, yogurt, etc.) or with the drink with the meal;

- If you still feel thirsty, use a slice of lemon to moisten your lips, add an ice cube with possibly some lemon juice for an even fresher taste and increase saliva production (corresponds to 15 ml of water). You can also use a small portion of the fruit that you could freeze for this. You can also rinse the mouth with water.
- The use of humidifiers can also be a tool to prevent dry mouth and provide the necessary refreshment in hot weather.

Top 15 kidney-friendly nutrition for people with kidney problems

1. Red pepper

- 75 grams of red pepper = 1 mg of sodium, 88 mg of potassium, 10 mg of phosphorus

Red peppers have a low potassium value and have a lot of taste, but that is not the only reason why they fit well in a kidney-friendly diet. These tasty vegetables are an excellent source for vitamin C, vitamin A. Vitamin B6, folic acid and fiber. Red peppers are good for you because they contain lycopene, an antioxidant that protects you against cancer.

2. Cabbage

- 75 grams of green cabbage = 6 mg of sodium, 60 mg of potassium and 9 mg of phosphorus

Cabbage is a cruciferous vegetable and is packed with phytochemicals, chemical components in fruit or vegetables that neutralize free radicals before they can cause damage. Many phytochemicals are known to fight cancer and to support cardiovascular health.

Cabbage contains a lot of vitamin K, vitamin C, and fiber. It is also a good source of vitamin B6 and folic acid. It is low in potassium and inexpensive and is, therefore, an affordable addition to a kidney-friendly diet.

3. Cauliflower

- 75 grams of cooked cauliflower = 9 mg of sodium, 88 mg of potassium and 20 mg of phosphorus

Cauliflower, another cruciferous vegetable, is a good source of vitamin C, fiber and folate (one of the B vitamins, and in large quantities also called folic acid and vitamin B9). It is also full of indoles, glucosinolates, and thiocyanates - constituents that help the liver neutralize toxins that damage cell membranes and DNA.

4. Garlic

- 1 clove of garlic = 1 mg of sodium, 12 mg of potassium and 4 mg of phosphorus

Garlic helps to prevent plaque, lowers your cholesterol and reduces inflammation.

5. Onions

- 75 grams of onions = 3 mg of sodium, 116 mg of potassium and 3 mg of phosphorus

Onions are part of the basic flavorings in every kitchen, contain sulfur, and therefore give it its sharp odor. Although onions make some people shed tears, they are also rich in flavonoids, and in particular quercetin, a powerful antioxidant that helps fight heart disease and protects against various cancers. Onions are low in potassium and are a good source for chromium, a mineral that helps in carbohydrate, protein and fat metabolism.

6. Apples

- 1 medium apple with zest = 0 sodium, 158 mg of potassium and 10 mg

Apples are known to lower cholesterol, prevent constipation, protect against heart disease and reduce the risk of cancer. Apples are high in fiber and have many anti-inflammatory components. The slogan "Sweets healthy, eat an apple" seems to have a solid foundation.

7. Cranberries

- 75 grams of cranberry juice cocktail = 3 mg of sodium, 22 mg of potassium and 3 mg of phosphorus
- 40 grams of cranberry sauce = 35 mg of sodium, 17 mg of potassium and 6 mg of phosphorus
- 75 grams of dried cranberries = 2 mg of sodium, 24 mg potassium, and 5 mg phosphorus

These tasty berries are known to offer protection against bladder infection by preventing bacteria from sticking to the bladder wall. Similarly, cranberries protect the stomach from ulcer-causing bacteria, and protect your gastrointestinal tract and even help improve its health. It has also been found that cranberries help against cancer and heart disease.

8. Blueberries

- 75 grams of fresh blueberries = 4 mg of sodium, 75 mg of potassium and 7 mg of phosphorus

Blueberries contain many antioxidant phytonutrients called anthocyanidins, which give them their blue color. They are full of natural compounds that reduce inflammation. Blueberries are a good source of vitamin C, manganese (that keeps your bones healthy), and fiber. They can also help protect your brain against some of the effects of aging.

9. Raspberries

- 75 grams of raspberries = 0 mg of sodium, 93 mg of potassium and 7 mg of phosphorus

Raspberries contain a phytonutrient called ellagic acid that helps neutralize free radicals in the body and thus prevent cell damage. They also contain the flavonoids anthocyanins - antioxidants that give raspberries their red color. Raspberries are an excellent source for manganese, vitamin C, fiber and folate, a vitamin B. Raspberries can have properties that can prevent cancer cell growth and tumor formation.

10. Strawberries

- 75 grams (5 medium) fresh strawberries = 1 mg of sodium, 120 mg of potassium and 13 mg of phosphorus

Strawberries are full of two types of phenols: anthocyanins and ellagitannins. Anthocyanins give strawberries their red color and are powerful antioxidants that help protect the structure of body cells and prevent damage due to oxidation. Strawberries are full of vitamin C and manganese and are an excellent source of fiber. They are known to protect the heart and contain anti-cancer and anti-inflammatory properties.

11. Cherries

75 grams of fresh (sweet) cherries = 0 mg of sodium, 160 mg of sodium and 15 mg of phosphorus
Eating cherry daily helps prevent inflammation. They are also full of antioxidants and phytochemicals that protect the heart.

12. Red Grapes

- 75 grams of red grapes = 1 mg of sodium, 88 mg of potassium and 4 mg of phosphorus
Red grapes contain different flavonoids that give them their reddish color. Flavonoids prevent oxidation and reduce blood clots and thereby help protect against heart disease. Resveratol, a flavonoid contained in grapes, can also stimulate the production of nitrogen oxides; this helps relax the muscle cells in blood vessels and promote blood flow. These flavonoids also protect against cancer and prevent inflammation.

13. Protein

- 2 proteins = 7 grams of protein, 110 mg of sodium, 108 mg of potassium and 10 mg of phosphorus
Protein is pure protein and provides the highest amount of protein with all essential amino acids. Proteins fit well in a kidney-friendly diet because they contain less phosphorus than other proteins such as egg yolk or meat.

14. Fish

- 85 grams of wild salmon = 50 mg of sodium, 368 mg of potassium and 274 mg of phosphorus
Fish supplies high-quality protein and contains omega 3, an anti-inflammatory fat. These healthy fats in fish help to combat diseases such as heart disease and cancer. Omega 3 also helps in

lowering LDL cholesterol (the bad cholesterol) and in raising HDL, the good variant of cholesterol. Fish species high in omega 3 include Albine tuna, herring, mackerel, rainbow trout, and salmon.

15. Olive oil

- 1 tablespoon of olive oil = less than 1 mg of sodium, less than 1 mg of potassium and 0 mg of phosphorus

Olive oil is a great source of oleic acid, a fatty acid with an anti-inflammatory effect. The unsaturated acid in olive oil protects against oxidation. Olive oil is rich in polyphenols and antioxidants that prevent inflammation and oxidation.

Research shows that populations that use large amounts of olive oil instead of other oils are less likely to suffer from heart disease and cancer.

Virgin or extra virgin olive oil contains more antioxidants.

Tips to prevent kidney damage

Tips for a healthy lifestyle

Maintaining a healthy lifestyle sounds so simple, but it is sometimes so difficult. Below you can read what a healthy lifestyle is and how you can reduce the risk of kidney damage. Many of these recommendations will correspond to the lifestyle recommendations that are given for high blood pressure and diabetes, diseases that in themselves can lead to kidney damage.

Healthy food

Whoever eats according to the guidelines of the Voedingscentrum and also has a regular eating pattern, will feel nice and fit and also reduce the risk of kidney damage. Eat varied, not too much, less saturated fat, less salt, lots of vegetables, lots of fruit and enough bread.

Healthy weight

People who are overweight have an increased risk of kidney damage (and of other diseases such as diabetes and cardiovascular disease). It is, therefore, important to strive for a healthy weight. The Body Mass Index (BMI) is used worldwide to determine whether someone has a healthy weight. So check regularly how your BMI is doing.

Enough exercise

For your health, it is useful to moderate intensity for one hour daily exercise. That means that you have to breathe correctly, and your heart beats faster. Moving for half an hour does not have to be consecutive. Cycling twice for 15 minutes or walking ten times for 10 minutes is also possible.

Do not smoke

Smoking can damage the blood vessels in and towards the kidneys. It is, therefore, an important risk for kidney damage. Stopping smoking ensures that your health immediately jumps. And you notice it: your breathing improves, coughing becomes less, the condition goes up and smelling and tasting goes better.

Moderate drinking

For adult men and women, moderate drinking means on average no more than a standard glass per day. The benefits of drinking alcohol do not outweigh the disadvantages. That is why the advice is not to drink alcohol or at least not more than 1 glass per day. In any case, try to insert a number of alcohol-free days.

Use as little salt as possible

Using minimal salt is very important in preventing kidney damage. Salt can lead to high blood pressure, which is harmful to the kidneys. And salt is also directly harmful to the kidneys, especially if there is kidney damage. Protein loss in the urine - which is detrimental to the kidneys, heart and blood vessels - also decreases due to salt restriction.

Tips for eating less salt

Eating less salt can delay the worsening of kidney damage. But it can be challenging to reduce salt. Much of the salt that you get is already in the products when you buy them. And you may have to get used to the taste of eating less salt.

These tips help you eat less salt:

- Give yourself time to get used to it
- Choose unprocessed foods
- Do not add salt yourself
- Avoid salty seasonings
- Use herbs, spices, and seasonings such as onion and garlic
- Eat less salty bread meals
- Let someone else cook (sometimes)
- Avoid licorice, liquorice tea, minty Maroc tea, and star mix tea

1. Give yourself time to get used to it

Remember that it takes time to get used to a meal without salt. You have to get rid of the salty taste. This is only possible by consistently not using salt or salty seasonings. In the beginning, less salt food tastes mostly bland, but after a while, you will taste better, and you will find a lot of salt dirty.

2. Choose unprocessed food

Processed foods are products that the manufacturer has processed with salt or other flavorings. These products contain (a lot of) salt. Think of ready-made sauces and soups, and ready-made meals. Avoid processed meat, such as hamburgers, roulade, seasoned minced meat, and sausage. Also, do away with processed fish, such as marinated fresh fish, breaded (frozen) fish, steamed and smoked fish, and canned fish and pickled fish.

Therefore, choose unprocessed food: unprocessed meat, unprocessed chicken, unprocessed fish, and fresh vegetables or frozen vegetables. Season with herbs and spices if necessary.

Ask a butcher to prepare processed meat without salt, such as a low-sodium variant of processed meat like a roulade.

Choose vegetable preserves without added salt: look at the health food store or the supermarket diet

Cook extra portions and store them in the freezer, as an alternative to a salty ready-made meal.

Compare labels

Compare different brands and variants of food. The differences in the amount of salt are large. If you always choose the brand or variant with the least salt, your salt intake will decrease.

3. Do not add salt yourself

Do not add any more salt yourself when cooking. Place the salt pot far away so that you do not grab it automatically.

Also, do not use salt products with other names. Such as:

Celery salt, garlic salt, onion salt, Himalayan salt or Celtic sea salt. These contain just as much salt as common kitchen salt.

Dietary salt, half-salt and mineral salt contain much less sodium than ordinary salt. Potassium is in it instead. If you have a potassium limitation, these products are not a suitable alternative to salt.

Monosodium glutamate (E621): This is a flavor enhancer that contains sodium. It is also known as Chinese salt or Ve-tsin.

4. Avoid salty seasonings

Avoid the use of salty seasonings. For example, Maggi, bouillon cubes, soy sauce, scattering aroma, and soy sauce.

Sodium-limited variant

A sodium-limited version of many flavorings is also available. Ask about it at supermarkets or health food stores. Sodium-limited flavorings often contain potassium. Look at the label. Potassium is also listed as potassium chloride or E508. If you have a potassium restriction, then these sodium-restricted flavorings are not a suitable alternative.

5. Use herbs

Use fresh or dried garden herbs and spices to add flavor to your food.

Avoid ready-to-use spice mixes, ready-to-eat vegetable seeds and spice mixtures such as minced meat. Most of them consist of salt!

Traditional spice mixes such as meat, minced meat, and fish herbs contain salt. But there are also variants without salt for sale: you can often find them in the diet section of the supermarket.

There are many mixed herbs for sale without added salt. They are just in the spice box. Check the label for salt.

6. Eat less salty bread meals

Each slice of bread contains 0.35 grams of salt. Your salt intake decreases if you choose bread without salt. Bread without salt must be ordered from the bakery, or bake yourself.

You also eat less salt if you choose spreads that contain less salt. The siege below contains less salt than 1 slice of regular 48+ Gouda cheese or 1 portion of normally salted meats:

- cheese with less salt (25% or 33% less salt)
- Emmental or Gruyere cheese
- MonChou, cottage cheese
- Mozzarella
- Swiss stray cheese
- slightly salted meats: roast beef, slightly salted smoked meat, fricandeau, turkey breast, chicken breast
- peanut butter
- dairy spread
- sandwich spread, vegetable spread
- fruit: strawberry, apple/pear slices, banana slices
- raw vegetables: radish, cress, cucumber slices
- sweet toppings, such as jam

7. Have someone else cook (sometimes)

Do you not want to or cannot cook without salt? Then there are several other good options. Do not opt for ready-made meals from the supermarket, the butcher or the greengrocer. These contain a lot of salt. Below are some good alternatives.

Open table

Many nursing homes offer residents the option of eating a hot meal for a fee. Diet meals are possible. You must be able to come to the nursing home yourself.

Meals on Wheels
Table-cover-you is a service for the elderly and the long-term sick. You will receive the complete main meals delivered to your home. That can be a hot meal or a cooled meal that you need to heat. Diet meals are possible. Ask about the table at the home care institution in your municipality.

Frozen meals at home
Some organizations deliver frozen meals to order on demand. Diet meals are often also possible.

Tips for eating less saturated fat

People with kidney damage often also have high blood pressure. And an increased amount of fats in the blood, such as cholesterol and triglycerides. High blood pressure and high cholesterol increase the risk of cardiovascular disease.

Eating less saturated fat and more unsaturated fat reduces your risk of cardiovascular disease.

Tips for eating less saturated fat

Choose soft margarine or soft low-fat margarine with at least 50% polyunsaturated fatty acids.

For baking, roasting, and deep-frying, choose soft or liquid fats with a high percentage of unsaturated fat or oil.

Eat fish once a week in particular fatty fish, such as salmon, sardines, and mackerel. Smoked fish contains much more salt than fresh fish.

Limit the use of foods in which saturated fat is hidden, such as cakes, chocolate, and snacks. In some situations, for example, with a poor nutritional status, your dietician may advise you to use these foods temporarily.

Unsaturated fat is better

Fats consist of fatty acids. There are two types: saturated fatty acids and unsaturated fatty acids. Also: saturated fat and unsaturated fat.

Saturated fat raises blood cholesterol. This increases the risk of cardiovascular disease.

Unsaturated fat helps prevent barrels from narrowing. Narrowed and blocked vessels cause cardiovascular disease. Unsaturated fat helps prevent this.

Foods with lots of unsaturated fat are okay:
- all types of oil (including olive oil)
- soft margarine
- liquid cooking fat
- soft low-fat margarine
- nuts
- Fatty fish

Note: some bread spreads are enriched with potassium. These are less suitable if you have a potassium restriction.

Foods with a lot of saturated fat are wrong:
- butter
- margarine in a package
- full-fat cheese
- whole milk products
- whipped cream
- fat meat
- coconut
- chocolate
- pastries and snacks

Tips against food infections

Good hygiene is always important, even with food that looks good, smells good and tastes great. Because that too can contain bacteria that make you sick.

Tips against food infections

Only eat cooked foods

Avoid cross-contamination

Keep prepared products limited

Avoid products with listeria bacteria

Be careful with raw products and soft ice cream

If you are going on holiday abroad, then additional measures apply. The simpler the circumstances and the warmer the climate, the greater the chance that you will contract a food infection.

1. Only eat cooked foods

Make sure that meat, chicken, and egg are well-cooked before you eat them. The high temperature at which food cooks also kills bacteria.

2. Avoid cross-contamination

During cooking, avoid any contact between raw foods and prepared foods (especially meat, fish and chicken). Otherwise, you contaminate a cooked dish with new bacteria.

Take a clean dish towel and kitchen towel daily. Wash it at 60 ° C.

3. Do not store prepared products for too long

You can store prepared products in the fridge for a maximum of 24 hours, provided it is 5 ° C or cooler in the fridge. If the temperature is higher, the food cannot be stored for as long.

4. Avoid products with listeria bacteria

Avoid foods that contain listeria bacteria:
- Raw milk cheese
- Pre-packaged smoked fish
- Raw animal products

5. Avoid raw products and soft ice cream

Avoid products from raw fish and raw meat, such as shrimps and tartar and products with raw egg (such as desserts and meringues) and with soft ice cream.

Tips against constipation

Constipation is also called slow bowel movements or constipation. It means that pooping is difficult. Blockage can occur as a side effect of certain medicines, such as phosphate binders and iron preparations. But constipation can also be due to a shortage of dietary fiber, a fluid restriction or too little exercise. Constipation is also a side effect of dialysis, in particular, peritoneal dialysis (abdominal flushing).

Your lifestyle has a lot of influence on your bowel movements. These tips can help against clogging:

- Eat enough dietary fiber
- Eat regularly
- Go to the toilet if you feel an urge
- Keep moving
- Drink enough (unless you have a fluid restriction)

1. Eat enough dietary fiber

Eat foods rich in dietary fiber. Which are:

- Rye bread, wholemeal bread, and brown bread
- Wholemeal products such as oatmeal, muesli, wheat flakes
- Whole wheat pasta, brown rice,
- Vegetables, raw vegetables, fruit (preferably with peel) and potatoes
- Dried and soaked dried fruits such as plums, apricots, tutti-frutti, and raisins
- Nuts, peanuts
- Legumes, such as brown and white beans, capuchins and lentils

Note: many of these foods are rich in potassium. Keep this in mind if you have a potassium restriction.

2. Eat regularly

Eat regularly. That keeps the intestines moving. It is a personal choice whether you eat something 3 times a day or 5 times. But it is important that your eating rhythm is about the same every day. And at least don't skip your breakfast. Eating at the start of the day stimulates your intestines.

3. Go to the toilet if you feel an urge

Listen to your body. Go to the toilet immediately if you feel an urge. If you stop it, the poo will get hard.

4. Keep moving

Try to move more, as far as possible in your situation. Walking helps better against constipation than cycling or swimming.

5. Drink enough

Do you have no moisture restriction? Then drink 2 to 2.5 liters of fluid per day. Too little moisture can cause dry, hard stools.

Stop smoking: 10 pitfalls and tips.

Pitfall 1. Arrive by weight

The fear of arriving is one of the most important obstacles for people to quit smoking. That fear is partly justified because nicotine speeds up metabolism and by stopping, many smokers gain a few kilos. If this is a tricky issue for you, consider in advance how you can counteract weight gain as much as possible.

Simultaneous dieting and quitting smoking are often discouraged because for most people; it is too much of a good thing. But stopping smoking is another great time to take a closer look at your entire lifestyle. Make a plan in advance in your head how you will handle extra kilos. The one takes a few extra pounds for granted. Another intends to get rid of the kilos in half a year, and another person prevents weight gain by exercising more in advance or paying extra attention to his eating habits.

Pitfall 2. Feeling hungry

Nicotine inhibits appetite and stoppers will get more appetite for food. Stopping smoking also improves your taste and smell, so you can get more hunger. Before you stop, look for recipes that fill well, but that will not make you arrive, for example, meal salads and soups. A soup beforehand will satisfy the worst appetite.

Pitfall 3. Unhealthy snuffers

If you already know that you will fall prey to snails, make sure you have a plan for the difficult moments. Usually, the quiet evenings in front of the tube or with a book are the most difficult. It is almost impossible never to have a blow, but try to limit the amount of snacks or simply do not bring them home. Preferably look for spicy snacks, because you often have enough of these. For example, radishes, cauliflower florets or carrots with garlic dip or tzatziki are very suitable for temporarily reducing the need for a cigarette.

Pitfall 4. Fall into old habits

With smoking addiction, the habit is sometimes more stubborn than physical addiction. Often not all cigarettes a person smokes a day are needed to meet the physical addiction. Cigarettes can also be lit out of habit, for example, because it is a break or because you are going to drink coffee. For example, if you are used to smoking a cigarette while studying or doing household chores as a moment of rest, try to arrange this break in a different way. Before you stop smoking, try to list those habitual cigarettes and think about how you can capture those moments with other activities.

Pitfall 5. Keep cigarettes and ashtrays

Stopping smoking is hard enough. Don't make it harder on yourself by storing your cigarettes, lighters, and ashtrays. It is better to throw them all away so that you are not reminded of smoking. A partner who also smokes can also hamper your stop-smoking attempt for the same reason, so, therefore, it is advisable for you to quit together. That makes it easier for both of you.

Pitfall 6. Reduce smoking

Some people think it helps to reduce smoking first before you stop. Yet this often does not seem to work! Decreasing alone does not usually improve your health because even small amounts of smoke are already harmful. In addition, people with a disability often go for longer with one cigarette, and they also breathe in the smoke deeper, which ultimately results in almost as many unhealthy substances. It is also very difficult to reduce smoking alone. That is why the tip is to stop smoking cold turkey.

Pitfall 7. Afraid of concentration problems and unrest

Many smokers are afraid of concentration problems and unrest. They are afraid of not being able to work, write or sleep properly. Concentration problems are indeed part of the withdrawal symptoms of smoking. You can avoid these in the first few weeks by using nicotine substitutes such as chewing gum or plasters and gradually reducing them.

Pitfall 8. Use unprepared anti-smoking medication

Anti-smoking medication such as Zyban or Nortrilen is sometimes prescribed by doctors. These antidepressants are used in small doses as an anti-smoking pill. Some smokers benefit, but they are relatively heavy drugs, with the risk of side effects and in the case of Zyban allergic reactions. So think carefully about what you might use as an aid.

Pitfall 9. Not knowing where to relax

Most smokers cannot escape a tense feeling in the first few weeks, especially those who associate smoking with moments of rest or who relieve stress must find other ways to relax. It is very important to complete this search process before you stop smoking. In the first days of quitting smoking, the stress of quitting is added. And if you're used to relieving stress with a cigarette, you literally don't know where to look. Walking outside, working out, visiting a sauna, a massage, a hot bath, cinema or a good book; make an inventory in advance where you as a brand new non-smoker can get the best relaxation and distraction from and start practicing with it.

Pitfall 10. Not having a good incentive

Before you stop smoking, think about what is an important motivation for you to quit smoking. For some, that is the example for the children, for others, maintaining beautiful skin and for third, healthy lungs. Think of the motivation in the difficult moments, and maybe it can help you to get through the difficult moment.

90+ recipes

Ciabatta

Ingredients
- 15 g fresh yeast
- 700 g flour (type 405)
- 5 tbsp milk (1.5% fat)
- 2 tbsp olive oil
- 20 g sea salt
- 200 g fine wheat wholemeal flour
- some flour to work

Preparation
Prepare the batter the night before: Dissolve 5 g of yeast in 250-260 ml of lukewarm water in a bowl and let stand for 10 minutes.
Sift 350g of flour. Stir with a wooden spoon for 5 minutes until sticky dough is formed.
Cover the bowl with cling film and leave for 12 hours at room temperature.
Prepare the main dough the next day: Dissolve the remaining yeast in the warm milk and let stand for 10 minutes.
Add 250 ml of water (room temperature), olive oil and starter dough and knead with the dough hooks of the hand mixer.
Mix salt with remaining flour and fine wholemeal flour and gradually add to the dough, kneading for about 4 minutes.
Sprinkle the work surface with flour, put the ciabatta dough on it and knead it vigorously by hand for 2-3 minutes.

Lightly oil a bowl. Add ciabatta dough, turn over and cover with cling film. Leave at room temperature for about 1 1/2 hours. The gone ciabatta dough should be very airy, sticky and elastic.
Carefully pull with your hand.
Generously dust 2 pieces of baking paper with flour and place the loaves of bread on top.
Press, in each case a few "dimples" with the fingertips. Dust 2 kitchen towels with flour on one side and cover the ciabatta loaves with them. Let it go for 1 1/2 hours.
Place 2 ciabatta loaves with baking paper on a baking tray and sprinkle the oven wall with a little water. Bread in the pre-heated oven at 250 ° C (circulating air: 220 ° C, gas: 4-5) bake for about 20-25 minutes and let cool on an oven rack. Bake the remaining ciabatta loaves in the same way.

-

Rice with stir-fried chicken fillet and bok choy

Ingredients
- 200 g chicken fillet
- 1 shrub bok choy
- 1 red pepper
- 200 g of rice
- 2 tbsp oil
- 2 tbsp curry
- 1 clove of garlic, chopped
- ½ red pepper, chopped without seeds
- 1 cup of crème Fraiche

Preparation
Cut the chicken into cubes. Clean the bok choy and cut the stems and leaves into strips of approximately 2 centimeters. Clean the bell pepper and cut it into small strips.
Prepare the rice according to the instructions on the package. In the meantime, heat the oil in a wok (or frying pan) and stir-fry the chicken until brown, then fry the garlic and chili.

Sprinkle the chicken with the curry and stir in the bok choy and bell pepper. Stir fry the whole for another 5 minutes.

Drain the rice well.

Stir the crème fraîche into the meat and vegetable mixture and stir-fry until everything is thoroughly hot.

Season the dish with pepper.

-

Amaranth muesli bars

<u>Ingredients</u>
- 50 g flaked almonds
- 40 g sunflower seeds
- 25 g peanut kernel (unsalted)
- 50 g 5-grain cereal flakes
- 30 g puffamaranth
- 1 tsp cinnamon
- 25 g sultanas
- 1 pinch salt
- 75 g butter
- 50 g cane sugar
- 4 tbsp liquid honey

<u>Preparation</u>
Put almond flakes, sunflower seeds, peanut kernels, cereal flakes, amaranth and dates in a bowl. Add cinnamon, sultanas, and salt and mix well.

Melt the butter in a saucepan over low heat. Add sugar and honey and bring to a boil over medium heat with constant stirring.

Add hot sugar mixture to the remaining ingredients and mix thoroughly with a wooden spoon. Lay out a springform pan (24 cm) with baking paper and add the mixture.

Press firmly and bake in a pre-heated oven at 180 ° C (circulating air: not recommended, gas: stage 2-3) for about 25 minutes. Allow cooling completely, release from the mold and cut into triangles.

175

Red currant jelly

Ingredients

- 1800 g red currants
- 500 g gelling sugar made from whole cane sugar 3: 1
- 12 coffee beans

Preparation

Wash currants and drain well.

Using a fork, brush the berries off the stems.

Place the berries in a large saucepan and add 150 ml of water. Cover the berries and bring them to a boil for about 30 minutes, stirring occasionally.

Lay out a fine sieve with a kitchen towel and hang over a pot. Pour berries and juice into the strainer and drain thoroughly for 5-6 hours. Meanwhile, wash 4 screw jars (400 ml each) and rinse the appropriate lid with boiling water and drain headfirst on a kitchen towel.

Measure 1.2 l of juice. Put in a saucepan with gelling sugar and mix.

Place the coffee beans in a kitchen towel, seal with kitchen yarn and add to the pot with the juice.

Bring the juice to a boil while stirring constantly.

When boiling, boil off with a foam trowel, and boil the juice bubbly for 4 minutes.

Remove the coffee bean bag.

Fill the prepared glasses with hot liquid and close with the lids. Leave for about 5 minutes, then stand upright again.

Raspberry jelly with mint

Ingredients

- 2 kg raspberries
- 4 stems mint
- 500 g gelierzucker 3: 1

Preparation

176

Read raspberries, rinse carefully in a sieve and drain well.

Place the berries in a large saucepan and add 150 ml of water. Cover the berries and bring to a boil. Let them simmer for about 30 minutes, stirring occasionally.

Lay out a fine sieve with a kitchen towel and hang over a pot. Strain berries and juice and drain thoroughly for 5-6 hours. Meanwhile, 4 screw jars (400 ml each) and rinse the appropriate lid with boiling water and drain headfirst on a kitchen towel.

Wash mint and shake dry. Pluck leaves.

Measure 1.2 l of juice. Put the gelling sugar in a saucepan and stir.

Bring the juice to a boil while stirring constantly.

When boiling boil off foam with a skimmer and boil the juice while stirring bubbly for 4 minutes.

Add mint and cook for another 30 seconds.

Fill the prepared glasses with hot liquid and cover with lids. Leave for about 5 minutes.

-

Blackberry and elderberry jelly

Ingredients
- 1400 g blackberry
- 600 g elderberries
- 500 g gelierzucker 3: 1
- ½ lemon

Preparation
Wash the blackberries and drain well.

Rinse elderberries, drain well and pluck from the stems.

Put all the berries in a saucepan and add 150 ml of water.

Cover slowly and bring to a boil. Simmer covered for about 30 minutes, stirring gently from time to time.

Lay out a fine sieve with a kitchen towel and hang over a pot. Put the berries in the sieve and drain thoroughly for about 5-6 hours. In the meantime, rinse 3 screw jars (400 ml each) with matching lids with boiling water and drain upside down on a kitchen towel.

Measure a total of 1.2 l from the drained berry juice. Put the gelling sugar in the pot and bring to a boil, stirring constantly.

When cooking, remove the rising foam with a skimmer and let the juice boil for 4-6 minutes. Squeeze out the lemon. Stir 2 tablespoons of lemon juice under the jelly and cook for another 30 seconds.

Hot fill the liquid into the prepared glasses and close immediately. Leave for about 5 minutes, then stand upright again.

-

Papaya and orange jam

Ingredients

- 1000 g papaya (2 papayas)
- 500 g oranges (3 oranges)
- 500 g gelierzucker 3: 1

Preparation

Peel papayas, cut in half and remove the seeds.

Cut the pulp into small cubes.

Peel oranges so thick that all white skin is removed.

Remove the pulp from the skins and add to the papaya cubes. Squeeze the skins thoroughly and mix the juice with the fruit. All together should weigh about 1.3 kg.

Add the jelly sugar, mix everything thoroughly and leave for about 2 hours. In the meantime, rinse 4 screw jars (400 ml each) with matching lids with boiling water and drain upside down on a kitchen towel.

Put the papaya and orange mix in a saucepan, bring to a boil while stirring and then boil for 4 minutes while stirring.

Fill the prepared glasses with hot liquid and cover with lids. Leave for about 5 minutes, then stand upright again.

-

Carrot drink

Ingredients

- 2 small cloves of garlic
- 800 g bunch of carrots
- 1 bunch smooth parsley
- ½ lemon
- 1 tsp rapeseed oil

Preparation

Peel garlic cloves.

Thoroughly wash carrots and cut off the ends.

Wash the parsley and shake dry. Squeeze lemon half off.

Juice garlic and 6 carrots in the juicer.

Add parsley and remaining carrots to the juicer and juice.

Mix carrot drink with about 2 tablespoons of lemon juice and the rapeseed oil and enjoy immediately.

Spicy apple and pineapple juice

Ingredients

- 600 g apples (3 apples)
- ¼ pineapple (about 250 g of pulp)
- 25 g ginger root (1 piece)
- ½ lime

Preparation

Wash apples and cut small.

Peel the pineapple, remove the hard core and cut the pulp into large pieces.

Peel ginger and dice roughly. Squeeze out the lime.

Add apples, pineapple, and ginger to a juicer and juice. Season with lime juice and enjoy as quickly as possible.

Green fruit packets

Ingredients

- 200 g green seedless grapes
- 2 kiwis
- 300 g green-colored pears (2 green-colored pears)
- 300 g small melon (e.g. galia, 0.5 small melons)
- 8 g ginger (1 piece)
- 1 cinnamon stick
- 4 cardamom pods
- 4 tbsp maple syrup

Preparation

Wash the grapes, drain in a colander, pluck from the stems and cut in half.

Peel and slice the kiwis.

Wash pears, quarter, core and cut into slices.

Core melon with a teaspoon, cut into slices and peel.

Ginger peel and finely chop. Break the cinnamon stick into 4 small pieces.

From the baking paper cut 4 pieces of about 35x25 cm each.

Divide grapes, kiwi, pears and melon and ginger into 4 portions and put 1 serving in the middle of 1 piece of baking paper.

Add 1 piece of cinnamon stick and 1 cardamom pod and dribble 1 tbsp of maple syrup.

Fold the baking paper into small packets and close.

Cook in a preheated oven at 180 ° C (circulating air: 160 ° C, gas: stage 2-3) for about 15-20 minutes. Put on a plate, open slightly and serve.

Strawberry papaya drink

Ingredients

- 2 stems mint
- 250 g strawberries
- 2 kiwis
- 400 g papaya (1 papaya)

Preparation

Wash the mint, shake dry, peel off the leaves and set aside.

Wash strawberries carefully, drain on kitchen paper, clean, chop and place in a tall container. Puree with a hand blender and strain into 2 glasses.

Peel kiwis, halve, dice and place in a tall container. Purée with the hand blender and place gently with a spoon on the strawberry puree.

Halve the papaya and remove the seeds with a spoon. Remove the pulp from the skin, chop it roughly and puree with the hand blender. Carefully pour into jars, garnish with mint and serve immediately.

-

Orange bulgur

Ingredients
- 100 g bulgur
- 300 g large organic orange (250-1 large organic orange)
- ½ tl rapeseed oil
- 125 g small apples (1 small apple)
- 125 g small pears (1 small pear)
- 100 g grapes
- 1 fresh fig
- 125 g small bananas (1 small banana)
- ½ lime
- 2 tsp maple syrup

Preparation

Put bulgur in a bowl. Brew with 100 ml of boiling water and allow to swell for about 5 minutes.

Meanwhile, wash orange, rub dry and finely rub the skin. Halve orange, squeeze out and measure 120 ml of juice. Mix the juice, peel and rape oil with a fork under the swollen bulgur.

Wash the apple, pear, grapes, and fig and pat dry. Quarter a pear and apple. Cut the grapes in half and remove them if necessary, peel the banana. Cut all fruits into bite-sized pieces.

Squeeze half the lime and stir the juice in a small bowl with the maple syrup. Pour over the fruits, mix everything and leave to soak for 8-10 minutes. Serve with the orange bulgur and serve.

-

Artichoke cream on corn waffles

Ingredients
- 120 g small tomatoes (3 small tomatoes)
- 220 g Artichoke bottoms (can, drained weight)
- 5 g ground almonds (1 tsp)
  - salt
  - pepper
- 4 stems basil
- 2 corn waffle

Preparation
Wash the tomatoes, cut out the stems into a wedge shape.
2 quarters tomatoes; remove seeds and cut into 5 mm cubes.
Drain 3 artichoke bottoms, then cut into 1 cm pieces. Puree the half in a tall container with a hand blender.
Mix the artichoke puree with artichoke pieces, diced tomatoes and ground almonds. Season with salt, pepper and leave for 10 minutes.
Rinse the basil, shake dry and peel off the leaves. Put some aside for garnish, cut the rest into fine strips.
Stir under the artichoke cream, season with salt and pepper again and spread on the corn waffles. Garnish with basil leaves and serve.

-

Oat and pine nut crunchies

Ingredients
- 75 g pine nuts (or almonds)
- 250 g hearty oatmeal
- 2 tsp cinnamon
- 1 pinch salt

182

- 50 ml honey
- 50 ml maple syrup
- 2 tbsp rapeseed oil
- 50 g dried cherries

Preparation

Chop pine nuts, place in a bowl with the oatmeal. Add cinnamon and salt and mix everything.

Mix the honey, maple syrup and oil in a saucepan and bring to the boil while stirring.

Carefully lift with a wooden spoon under the mixture of flakes.

Lay out a baking sheet with baking paper and spread the mixture of flakes on it.

Bake in a preheated oven at 125 ° C (circulating air: 110 ° C, gas: stage 1-2) for approx. 1 1/4 hours, turning carefully 2 to 3 times.

Remove from the oven and allow to cool completely. Then mix the crunchies with the dried cherries. Fill in an airtight sealable glass; That's how the crunchies last for about 3 weeks. Remove by the portion.

Mango and raspberry cocktail

Ingredients
- 350 g ripe mango (1 ripe mango)
- 200 g pink grapefruit (1 pink grapefruit)
- 2 stems mint
- 150 g raspberries
- mineral water at will
- also: ice cubes

Preparation

Wash the mango and peel with a peeler. Slice the pulp from the stone and dice it.

Halve the grapefruit and squeeze it out.

Wash mint, shake dry, peel off leaves and cut into thin strips.

183

If necessary, gently rinse the raspberries, drain, and place with the mango cubes and grapefruit juice in a tall container. Puree with a hand blender and mix until foamy. Add ice cubes to glasses, fill with mineral water as desired and garnish with mint strips.

-

Melons and spinach juice

Ingredients
- 350 g small honeydew melon (0.5 small honeydew melons)
- 250 g young tender spinach leaves
- 1 piece cinnamon stick (about 1 cm)
- nutmeg
- also: ice cubes

Preparation
Core the melon with a teaspoon. First cut the melon into slices, then cut the flesh from the shell and chop it roughly.
Clean the spinach and wash thoroughly in a bowl of water. Repeat the water several times until it stays clear.
Scrape thin strips off the cinnamon stick with a small sharp knife. Express the spinach lightly; move a small leaflet and a small stalk for the garnish. Juice the rest with the melon in a juicer and pour ice cubes into a glass. Garnish with some nutmeg, garnish with cinnamon and possibly the spinach and enjoy immediately.

-

Baguette

Ingredients
- 250 g wheat flour type 550
- 225 g whole-wheat flour
- 15 g fresh yeast
- 12 g salt (2 tsp)
- 1 tbsp rapeseed oil

Preparation

On the eve of the pre-dough, put 125 g wheat flour and 75 g wheat wholegrain flour in a bowl. Break in 10 g of yeast and add 250 ml of lukewarm water.

Knead with the dough hook of the hand mixer for 1 minute. Cover well with cling film and let it rest for at least 12 hours at room temperature.

The next day, add the remaining flour and remaining whole wheat flour with salt in a bowl and in the middle of a depression. The remaining yeast crumbles in. Add 125 ml of lukewarm water and let rest for 10 minutes.

Add the dough to the other ingredients in the bowl and knead with the kneading hook of the hand mixer for 4 minutes.

Place the dough on a floured surface and knead for another 10 minutes by hand, possibly adding some flour until the dough no longer sticks to the hands.

Add oil to a bowl and turn the dough ball in it to wet the surface. Cover with cling film and leave at room temperature for 1 1/2 hours until the volume has doubled.

Lightly knead the dough together and form into an elongated loaf. Let it go for another 60 minutes.

Place the piece of dough on the floured work surface and quarter.

Bring the pieces of dough together by pressing lightly and rolling them in baguette sticks (about 25 cm in length).

Place the baguette pieces of dough on a baking tray covered with baking paper and leave to stand covered with a floured kitchen towel for 40 minutes.

Carve the baguettes diagonally several times with a very sharp knife. Bake in a preheated oven at 220 ° C (circulating air 200 ° C, gas: stage 3-4) on the second rail from below for 30-35 minutes.

Allow baguettes to cool on the oven rack before serving.

-